SKILLS FOR SOCIAL WORK PRACTICE

SKILLS FOR SOCIAL WORK PRACTICE

EDITED BY KEITH DAVIES
AND RAY JONES

 palgrave

First published 2016 by
PALGRAVE

Palgrave in the UK is an imprint of Macmillan Publishers Limited, registered in England, company number 785998, of 4 Crinan Street, London, N1 9XW.

Palgrave Macmillan in the US is a division of St Martin's Press LLC, 175 Fifth Avenue, New York, NY 10010.

Palgrave is a global imprint of the above companies and is represented throughout the world.

Palgrave® and Macmillan® are registered trademarks in the United States, the United Kingdom, Europe and other countries.

ISBN 978–1–137–39026–4

This book is printed on paper suitable for recycling and made from fully managed and sustained forest sources. Logging, pulping and manufacturing processes are expected to conform to the environmental regulations of the country of origin.

A catalogue record for this book is available from the British Library.

A catalog record for this book is available from the Library of Congress.

Library of Congress Cataloging-in-Publication Data

Davies, Keith, 1955- author.
  Skills for social work practice / Keith Davies, Ray Jones.
    pages cm
  Includes index.
  ISBN 978-1-137-39026-4 (pbk.)
  1. Social service—Practice.   2. Social workers.   I. Title.
  HV10.5.D386 2015
  361.3'2—dc23   2015033215

Printed in China

To our students, service users and carers and to the late Professor Olive Stephenson, all of whom have encouraged and inspired us. Special thanks to Professor Hilary Tompsett for her invaluable expertise and support.

CONTENTS

LIST OF FIGURES AND TABLES

Figures

Tables

FOREWORD

The acquisition and development of skills for social work practice is as critically re-examined today as it has been during the long history of social work practice and education. I am delighted to welcome this timely new book designed for student social workers and social work practitioners, particularly those reviewing their skills for the Assessed and Supported Year in Employment (ASYE) first introduced in September 2012. It will also be of value for educators in academic and practice settings including practice educators.

Skills, as described by the Social Work Reform Board (2010, 2012) and in reviews commissioned on social work and education (Munro, 2011; Narey, 2014; Croisdale-Appleby, 2014), are part of social work professional behaviours, attitudes, knowledge and values. The frameworks outlining the skills required to meet professional and regulatory standards now include the College of Social Work's Professional Capabilities Framework (PCF) (2012) and the Health and Care Professions Council's Standards of Proficiency (SoPs) (2012). The challenge is how to help the development of key skills that can be assessed fairly without being reduced to checklists of activities and that will enable an emerging social worker to adapt and use them in changing contexts, and within different cultures, practice settings and roles. The social work profession has in recent years seen an increasingly fast turnover of policies, structures and drivers having an impact on professional practice and morale, while also challenging the best ways to attract and educate future social workers. It is timely, therefore, that this book is written to ensure the enduring and vital components of social work practice skills are identified, while bringing them up to date in the current terminology and landscape.

This book encompasses the following:

- different kinds of skills, for example, for communication (interpersonal and written) and relationship building, reflective practice, assessment and planning, and in using practice methods;

- skills for working in a wide range of practice-related contexts, including with service users and carers, in inter-professional practice, working with resistance and in leadership roles;

- some important areas of principles required for the proper exercise of skills, both ethical (including cultural competence) and legal.

The skill sections have been specifically linked with the domains of the PCF and the SoPs in order to make connections for lifelong professional development.

This book is written by a group of authors who have been at the forefront of providing high-quality social work education in local partnerships and engaged in national forums. Without exception, they are either registered social workers who are now based full time in higher education, current social work practitioners simultaneously teaching social work students, academics with specialist expertise (e.g. law) contributing to social work education, and/or current practice educators providing programmes of training and accreditation for other practice educators.

The learner-centred orientation of this book will be of particular benefit to readers who are seeking to strengthen and to extend their social work skills. It is particularly rich in examples from practice, evidence and research drawn from experience in social work practice, education and management, and engagement with service users and carers who have contributed to the review of the material, to the work described in Chapter 4 and to the inspiration and the motivation behind the writing of this book. With a very helpful introductory chapter, the set of chapters together provide, individually and collectively, a valuable new contribution to mastering professionalism in social work.

Hilary Tompsett, RSW (Registered Social Worker)
Emeritus Professor of Social Work, Kingston University & St George's, University of London
Chair, Joint University Council Social Work Education Committee (JUC SWEC) 2009–2014

References

Croisdale-Appleby, D. (2014) Re-visioning Social Work Education: An Independent Review, available at https://www.gov.uk/government/publications/social-work-education-review.

Health and Care Professions Council (2012) *Standards of Proficiency: Social Workers in England,* available at http://www.hpcuk.org/assets/documents/10003b08standards ofproficiency-socialworkersinengland.pdf.

Munro, E. (2011) *The Munro Review of Child Protection – Final Report: A Child-centred System,* available at http://www.education.gov.uk/munroreview/.

Narey, M. (2014) *Making the Education of Social Workers Consistently Effective,* https://www.gov.uk/government/uploads/system/uploads/attachment_data/file/287756/Making_the_education_of_social_workers_consistently_effective.pdf.

Social Work Reform Board (2010) *Building a Safe and Confident Future: One Year on.* London: Social Work Reform Board, available at www.education.gov.uk/swrb (now DfE archive).

Social Work Reform Board (2012) *Building a Safe and Confident Future: Maintaining Momentum*. London: Social Work Reform Board, available at www.education.gov.uk/swr (now DfE archive).

TCSW (2012) Professional Capabilities Framework, available at http:/www.tcsw.org.uk.

INTRODUCTION

This book is intended as a resource for social workers as they practise, alongside service users and carers, to enhance safety and well-being. It seeks to identify as clearly as possible which skills are associated with effective social work practices and how readers might take their own skill development forward.

Skills are often cited as one of three core components of effective social work practice in addition to knowledge and values (The College of Social Work, undated (a)), and it is accepted that skills not tempered by values and knowledge would be potentially abusive and misdirected. This book is necessarily about knowledge and values as well as skills and, indeed, skilled practice is understood as practice informed by both knowledge and values. However, the emphasis here is on skills where the term 'skills' refers to those actions (informed by theory, research, ethical principles, practice experience and reflection) by which social workers support service users in achieving safety and well-being.

Two key assumptions upon which the following chapters are founded are first that skills can be learnt and deepened through a variety of learning experiences and second that social workers continue to develop their skills throughout their working lives. Taking a lead from the Professional Capabilities Framework (PCF) (The College of Social Work, undated (b)) which describes a process of continuous learning and development across nine domains throughout a social worker's career, this book is intended for those engaged in social work at any point in their professional development. However, it may be especially useful to those in pre-qualifying training, qualifying training and the Assessed and Supported Year in Employment (ASYE) along with those working with them as educators. The approach is generic rather than specific to any particular practice specialism or service user group but it does relate most directly to an English practice context. Readers practising in Scotland, Northern Ireland and Wales should refer to the standards used by the relevant regulating bodies which may vary in detail, which can be found at the following addresses:

http://www.scswis.com/

http://www.rqia.org.uk/home/index.cfm

http://www.ccwales.org.uk/?force=1

The Context

This book appears at a time when social work practice is under intense scrutiny. Although this scrutiny has often been anxious, blaming and negative (see Jones, 2014, for a penetrating account of negative media and political attention), it has also been affirmative and driven by a positive, committed intention to support mature, intelligent, compassionate, assertive and determined practice (Munro, 2011). The Social Work Reform Board (SWRB) (2012) began the process of building a new framework for the development of professional skills.

As it noted, social work calls for a particular mix of analytical skills, insight, common sense, confidence, resilience, empathy and use of authority. Social workers are unlikely to develop these skills unless provided with high-quality education and training that continues throughout their careers; access to research and its practical applications; and high-quality working conditions with appropriate coaching, mentoring and supervision, and respect (p5).

Echoing this, Munro (2011) in her review of child protection placed a similarly positive emphasis on skill development. The review not only makes recommendations to enable social workers to exercise more professional judgement but also is concerned to improve their expertise. Building on the work of the Social Work Task Force (SWTF) and the Social Work Reform Board (SWRB), this review makes the case for radically improving the knowledge and skills of social workers from initial training to continuing professional development (Munro, 2011: 8–9)

The College of Social Work (TCSW) has been created with a remit to champion and stimulate the development of social work practice and, continuing the work of the SWRB, has developed and elaborated the PCF (TCSW, 2015 (c)) to support that process. At the same time, the Health and Care Professions Council (HCPC), a new regulator for social work, has identified a further framework of knowledge, values and skills in the Standards of Proficiency for Social Workers in England (SoPs) (2012). This book works with these frameworks to support the reader in evaluating and developing their skills. In each chapter, a 'Progress Check' feature identifies the key PCF domains and Standards of Proficiency which readers can use to measure their skill development.

Finally with regard to the contemporary interest in social work skills, two recent reports have focused on the quality of social work skills and social work education (Croisdale-Appleby, 2014; Narey, 2014). Knowledge and skills statements have also been developed for social workers in adults (Department of Health, 2015) and children's services (The Department for Education, 2014) following Narey's (2015) recommendations, whilst preparations have begun for a partnership approach to social work qualifying training which places an emphasis on practitioner–educators (DoE and DfE, 2015). This book is written with these developments very much in mind.

Structure and Contents

Since social work skills are multiple and interrelated, a choice has been made to cluster them into three main parts. The first part considers fundamental skills in communication and relationship building (Chapter 1 by Henderson and Mathew-Byrne), formal writing (Chapter 2 by Jones), ethical practice (Chapter 3 by Akhtar) and working with service users and carers (Chapter 4 by Skilton). Building on these foundational chapters, the second part focuses on skills involved in assessment (Chapter 5 by Hood), intervention skills using practice methods (Chapter 6 by Muleya), skills in drawing upon law in practice (Chapter 7 by Watson) and skilled use of reflection and supervision (Chapter 8 by Dicken and Van Graan). In the final part attention is paid to leadership (Chapter 9 by Davies and Ross), the development of skills in inter-professional practice (Chapter 10 by Barnes), and work with resistance (Chapter 11 by Gaskell-Mew and Lindsay).

The learner-centred orientation of this book will be of particular benefit to readers who actively seek to strengthen and to extend their social work skills. Each chapter follows a similar format and supports learning through the inclusion of case studies, reflective exercises, a check of progress in skills development in relation to the PCF, a chapter summary and indications for further reading. The structure will allow the book to be read either in its entirety and in sequence as a companion to a systematic learning process or in parts as the reader focuses on particular skills. It aims to respond to the needs of those asking such questions as: 'which key skills do I need to develop in order to practise successfully?' and 'how can I best learn and grow in these areas?' If the book supports social workers in any way in taking their skills forward, then it will have achieved its aim.

References

College of Social Work (undated (a)) *Understanding the Levels of the PCF*, available at http://www.tcsw.org.uk/uploadedFiles/PCF22NOVStudentLevelDescriptors.pdf, accessed 1 April 2015.

College of Social Work (undated (b)) *Understanding the PCF*, available athttp://www.tcsw.org.uk/understanding-the-pcf/, accessed 11 March 2015.

College of Social Work (undated (c)) *Practice Learning Guidance: 'Developing Skills for Practice' and 'Assessing Readiness for Direct Practice'*, available at http://www.tcsw.org.uk/uploadedFiles/TheCollege/_CollegeLibrary/Reform_resources/DevelopingSkillsReadiness(edref10).pdf, accessed 11 March 2015.

Croisdale-Appleby, D. (2014) Re-visioning Social Work Education: An Independent Review, https://www.gov.uk/government/uploads/system/uploads/attachment_data/file/285788/DCA_Accessible.pdf.

Department for Education (2015) *Knowledge and Skills for Child and Family Social Work*. London: Department for Education.

Department of Health (2015) *Knowledge and Skills Statement for Social Workers in Adult Services.* London: Department of Health.

Department for Education and Department of Health (2015) *Teaching Partnerships 2015–16: Invitation to Express Interest.* London: DoE, DfE.

Health and Care Professions Council (2012) *Standards of Proficiency for Social Workers in England.* London: HCPC.

Jones, R. (2014) *The Story of Baby P: Setting the Record Straight.* Bristol: Policy Press.

Munro, E. (2011) *The Munro Review of Child Protection: Final Report. A Child-centred System.* London: Department for Education.

Narey, M. (2014) *Making the Education of Social Workers Consistently Effective: Report of Sir Martin Narey's Independent Review of the Education of Children's Social Workers.* London: Department for Education.

Social Work Reform Board (2012) *Building a Safe and Confident Future: Maintaining Momentum. Progress Report from the Social Work Reform Board.* London: Department of Education.

1

DEVELOPING COMMUNICATION AND INTERVIEWING SKILLS

Kathleen Henderson and Jane Mathew-Byrne

Introduction

Effective communication skills are essential to becoming and being a social worker, used every day in professional practice and part of the repertoire of skills necessary for a professional. Good communication underpins all the skills discussed in this book, and this chapter provides a basis on which to draw when exercising them. It begins with examining communication skills for professional practice and aspects of professionalism for social workers. This includes consideration of what makes an effective communicator and what supports effectiveness, such as maintaining professional boundaries, and professional principles. The chapter explores the different contexts and roles in which social workers are required to exercise communication skills, for example, where they may have to exercise authority or make an assessment for services, and identifies core communication skills, including micro-skills that are likely to be used in an interview. By introducing a case study, we consider in more detail the stages for putting communication skills into practice: planning and structuring an interview, forming and maintaining relationships and taking a social history. Exercises to help with preparing oneself, self-reflection on communication and interviewing, and getting feedback from peers, service users and carers and other professionals follow. References are made throughout to the other chapters in this book with particular relevance to communication and interviewing skills, such as the chapters on written skills (2), working in partnership with service users and carers (4), assessment and planning (5), practice methods (6), reflective practice (8) and working with resistance (11).

Communication Skills for Professional Practice

While we use verbal and non-verbal communication in our non-professional everyday interactions with family, friends and colleagues, communication skills, when used in a professional context, involve 'learning to ask good questions, in ways likely to provide information that is both relevant and sufficiently detailed, and to watch for clues' (Trevithick, 2012: 154). Communication can take place in face-to-face interviews, telephone conversations and exchanges, meetings and reviews, and in writing. Written communication includes letters, case recordings and reports. Communication skills are also essential for developing and maintaining working relationships, for example, professional and inter-professional collaboration and supervision.

Communication as Part of Professionalism

As part of their professional education to become a qualified social worker, students will gain an understanding of what it means to belong to a profession and to act as a professional. Professionalism is perhaps not an easy concept and is best understood through participation in active experiential learning. Lishman (2009: 324) argues that skills development builds and establishes a professional culture that is an important element of professionalism: 'the establishment of a clear sense of professional identity is vital because it imparts confidence and role clarity, both of which are crucial when working closely with other professions'. The term 'new professionalism' used by Healy and Meagher (2004) recognises that sharing expertise and knowledge and drawing on the strengths of other people including service users, care providers and other professionals can add to professional understanding. Managing this engagement requires social workers to be able to listen to and discuss theirs and others' views effectively.

Social workers demonstrate professionalism and commitment to the profession by taking responsibility for their conduct and practice with service users and carers, and for their development throughout their professional life, both of which are supported through supervision. This will include reviewing their communication strengths, weaknesses and gaps. As representatives of the social work profession through their communication, they also safeguard its reputation.

What Makes a Social Worker an Effective Communicator?

Croisdale-Appleby (2014) identified that in order to become confident social work practitioners in any setting or role, social work students should be 'able to communicate with the service receiver and carer in order to diagnose and understand the situation and assess the risks involved; determine priorities in allocating limited resources; decide appropriate courses of action and manage that process'. They would also need to 'communicate effectively with professional colleagues who can contribute to those processes'. He also recognised that they will need 'the ability to exhibit resilience under conditions of high pressure' (2014: 15). This recognises the challenge of dealing with potentially sensitive subject matter, and the need for clarity of purpose and process, and skills to help people 'tell their story'.

A survey undertaken at Kingston University (2014), focusing on students, service users, carers and practice educators, explored the attributes of a social worker as an effective communicator.

Students thought that communication was a key skill, alongside reflection, time management and assertiveness. They felt that important personal attributes for being a good communicator included emotional resilience, integrity, empathy and self-awareness, as well as being knowledgeable (especially in relation to legislation, and their roles and responsibilities) and principled (with values such as being non-judgemental and passionate, maintaining professional boundaries and confidentiality and promoting advocacy and diversity).

Service users and carers valued relationship building primarily as a key element in good communication. They also identified other characteristics that aided communication, such as having clear professional boundaries, and the importance of integrity, empathy, the ability to develop relationships and a passion and commitment to the role. One young care leaver said, 'the best social worker I had was one who genuinely cared about me, and went the extra mile – doing little things like texting me and sending me a birthday card'.

Practice educators expected social work students to be able to transfer their knowledge and skills to different situations (i.e. to be flexible and adaptable) and to share information appropriately and clearly.

Social work lecturers also commented that, in order to be received well by those with whom social workers communicate, they need to pay attention to details, such as self-presentation, dress and posture in a meeting, and to show they are genuinely interested in others, putting aside their own concerns and focusing solely on the service user and their concerns.

Maintaining Professional and Personal Boundaries

Having clear personal and professional boundaries and knowing how to differentiate between them are crucial elements of our daily lives, although learning about them in a different context such as interviewing service users takes on a new meaning. The need to understand the differences between service users, colleagues and friends, that is, personal and professional relationships, is therefore crucial in supporting healthy professional boundaries as well as encouraging reflection about how we might be perceived.

Doel and Shardlow (2005) discuss the often paradoxical role of social work, where there is a need to be natural and engaging but at the same time professional and objective. This can be challenging for a student, however; understanding self-presentation and the possible subsequent impact this can have on the professional relationship is crucial. By practising and developing their professional style, students will not only increase their confidence/assertiveness but also their knowledge that work placements/situations will have different boundaries and expectations. Phillips (2013: 1) argues that to be assertive means recognising your own limitations and 'using our skills of attention, reasoning, awareness of feeling and behaviour to build the attributes of compassion'.

Principles of Good Social Work Communication

As part of social work practice and behaviour, communication by social workers is subject to regulatory standards of professional behaviour (as defined by the Health Professions Council), and good social work communication is 'informed by professional ethics, which include respect for culture, and a difficult combination of skills; being able to be authoritative and ask challenging questions' (Munro, 2011: 38).

The dilemma between being 'authoritative' while maintaining a constructive, compassionate and professional relationship is discussed in detail in the study of forming and maintaining relationships. Clarity about the role and purpose of the communication and involvement is important. Similarly, for a service user experiencing intervention in their lives, for example with decisions made about the removal of their children into the care system or depriving them of their liberty for their safety (under Mental Health legislation), the principle that they will also receive clear information about their rights and acknowledgement of the stress of the situation may be as important in accepting difficult outcomes.

Principles for effective communication also specifically include

- service user and carer participation (discussed in detail in Chapter 4);
- developing a trusting relationship;
- maintaining ethical and anti-oppressive practice (see also Chapter 3 alongside broader social work values including reliability and honesty).

Purposes and Kinds of Communication Skills and Micro-skills

Context and Purposes of Social Work Communication

You may be working as a student or practitioner in a local authority, a private, voluntary or independent agency, or in a service user or carer-led organisation. Your role may be very explicitly defined by the service or may be quite broad. Your contact with a service user/carer or other professional may also be a part of a longer-term case or a one-off referral/meeting. The reasons for your contact may therefore range from, for example, an initial assessment of what the problem or difficulty is, responding to a request for information/advice, investigating a specific allegation, intervening in a known crisis, discussing a specific service or eligibility for it or meeting to complete a form or application. Communication skills used in a professional conversation may be needed to inform, advise, clarify, question, probe and summarise while demonstrating sensitivity, genuineness, interest and responsiveness. Factors you may also need to consider include

- the situation – which may be complex, messy, distressing and/or confusing;

- the people – who may be pleased to meet you or may feel anxious, fearful, evasive, angry, hostile or resistant or all of these at times (Chapter 11 considers this in detail);

- attributes affecting communication capacity – such as sensory impairment (e.g. hearing or sight loss), cognitive impairment (e.g. from a stroke, learning difficulty, dementia), English not being the service user's or carer's first language or age-related special needs (e.g. talking to children);

- the urgency or level of risk attached to the referral or reason for contact;

- your own confidence, knowledge and experience.

All of this will affect how you prepare yourself and the kind of communication style or contact you plan. While initial contact is important, you may also be setting the scene for follow up, future contacts or intervention.

You may need to learn more about specialist skills such as communicating with children, using interpreters, relating to people with physical and learning disabilities and dealing with resistance, anger and hostility. For example, verbal communication alone is unlikely to meet the needs of children. The use of visual tools and playing with children, using art, stories and music, may be preferable methods. When communicating with a service user with a hearing loss, social workers need to negotiate the best method of communication. Options may include British sign language (BSL), using an interpreter, speaking to a representative or written communication.

What are the Core Communication Skills?

Skill, as defined by Shulman (2012: 6), refers to 'a specific behaviour that the worker uses in the helping process'; 'behaviour' may include the exercise of interpersonal, verbal and non-verbal observation, listening and assessment skills. Written and assessment skills are dealt with in more detail in other chapters (2 and 5).

Core communication skills used in interpersonal contact can be improved through use of techniques and awareness of one's own mannerisms and approach. Kadushin and Kadushin (2013: 151) describe techniques as 'conscious interventions'. Techniques include specific micro-skills such as active listening, use of minimum encouragers and of silence, and questioning, clarifying, reflecting, paraphrasing and summarising. These are explained later, integrating points on appropriate use of body language and the demonstration of empathy, which are also needed to be a 'skilled helper' (Egan, 2010).

Active Listening

This involves being alert to both the factual and the emotional content of what is being communicated. Social workers need to be sensitive to the social and cultural context of the service user, pick up on cues, avoid the dangers of pre-conceptions and premature judgements. Active listening can be very helpful in demonstrating empathy: it is important to try to understand what another person is feeling and gain a sense of what it is like to be in their world. Moss (2008: 87) draws the distinction between empathy and sympathy, stating that 'sympathy is an emotion or feeling that is generated within us by the misfortune of others' while empathy 'seeks to develop a more interactive relationship'.

Minimum Encouragers and Silence

These are used to enable the service user to talk; they include non-verbal minimal responses such as a nod of the head or positive facial expressions such as smiling, and verbal responses such as 'Uh-huh' and 'I hear what you're saying'. Equally important is learning to be comfortable with spaces in the conversation, and not being too quick to assume that verbal intervention is needed. If strong emotions are aroused in the speaker, they may need time to recover their composure or, if necessary, acknowledgement of the difficulty of the subject matter.

Open, Closed and Leading Questions

There are a range of different questions that can be used to elicit information such as open and closed questions, and probing. Closed questions help to elicit details such as age, ethnicity, family composition and social history while open questions invite more extensive answers and allow the service user to tell their story. Probing questions dig deeper to find out more about the other person. You can check if you are being given a full and accurate account by asking for more detail and checking against other information at hand. It is important to be aware that early assumptions can result in leading questions – leading the service user to agree with/confirm what you may have already decided.

Clarifying, Reflection, Paraphrasing and Summarising

Clarifying means using questions to ensure you understand what is being said so you are not confused and the client feels fully understood. It helps to gain an accurate picture of the situation and demonstrates the importance to the service user of the information they are sharing. Paraphrasing means using your own words to try and capture what you have heard, or as Trevithick (2012: 93) says, 'the essence of a person's statement is restated'. This is sometimes described as reflecting back on what you think you have heard. Summarising can be used throughout an interview and at the end to review the key points of a discussion and to bring a session to a close, by drawing together the main threads of the discussion.

Choice of Language, Appropriate Body Language and Cultural Awareness

The choice of words is important; avoiding jargon and using simple language helps. There is also a diversity of communication skills relating to cultural exchanges. For example, in some cultures, it is deemed disrespectful to maintain eye contact, but within Western culture it is quite the reverse. Poor eye contact can be viewed as lack of respect or not actively listening, therefore it is important to raise such points for critical reflection and learn from feedback (see also Chapters 3 and 8).

Communication skills can be learnt in the classroom; however feedback is essential. Without this the opportunity to develop and refine skills, and to find out how communication is received, is lost.

Putting Communication Skills into Practice in Interviews

Case Study 1.1 **The Gallagher family**

You are a social work student on placement at Sunhill Children and Families Team. You are on the duty desk when you receive a telephone referral from a school. The teacher informs you that she is very concerned about Jamie Gallagher who is seven years old.

▶

According to the teacher, since his return to school, following the summer holidays, Jamie has been tired and irritable, not able to focus on his work. The teacher states that 'He is often late in the morning, wearing stained clothes and complaining of being hungry. He has not completed any homework and is behind on his reading'.

The school is concerned about these issues as before the summer holidays Jamie was enthusiastic and a popular member of the class, and he was doing well academically. The teacher tried to talk to Jamie about what was happening at home, however he became very tearful saying that his mother was unwell and that she was sleeping all day. The teacher has not seen the parents, Mr and Mrs Gallagher, this term as Jamie is collected by his older brother after school. She has tried to telephone them but their phone appears to have been disconnected.

When you check on the system, you discover a number of facts – the family is known to the department, due to the parents' previous substance misuse. The family's cultural and religious background is Irish Catholic. Jamie has two siblings, aged twelve and five.

Reflective Exercise 1.1: **Planning an interview**

Your practice educator/manager suggests that you visit the Gallagher family at home to 'make an initial assessment'. You will need to enquire how things are for the family and see what support they may need. You need also to write a letter to the parents arranging to visit the family next week.

Initial preparation questions:

1 What seem to be the main issues? List them and prioritise if you can.

2 Who do you think will be your first communication contact?

3 What might you need to do to prepare yourself?

4 Who could assist you with this?

5 What aspects of being a professional do you need to think about?

Points to consider:

1 Is there anything you need to check before you visit?

2 How will you introduce yourself?

3 What is the purpose of your visit? You will need to explain who made the referral and summarise the concerns. What do you need to get out of the visit?

4 Which family members will you need to see?

5 How will you structure the interview?

6 How can you reassure the parents that you are here to help? Think carefully about your tone and choice of words, even preparing some forms of words.

7 How can you strike a balance between being supportive and professional?

8 How do you plan to end the interview?

After you have finished, think about how you would feel if you had a visit in relation to this kind of referral. Is there anything you would like to 'role play' or discuss in supervision first? Have you thought about what you will do if something unexpected happens (such as Mrs Gallagher behaving as if under the influence of substances)?

You may also want to think about how you would write a professional letter of introduction, drawing on the writing skills in Chapter 2.

Forming and Maintaining Relationships

The case study above reminds us that interviews do not happen in a vacuum, and of the importance of revisiting aspects of relationship in social work interviews. Practice examples are useful learning aids and the following scenario considers 'Susan', a newly qualified social worker, visiting the Gallagher family at home for the first time. The school raised concerns about their son Jamie's change in behaviour since returning to school following the summer holidays. Susan explains her role and wants to be seen as supportive and caring by the family – she achieves this by being very friendly and offering them many services. At a later date, the family feels very 'let down' by their 'friend' who has only provided them with one service. Susan realises she had inadvertently used the same communication skills of friendship which she employed as a youth club leader but which were not suitable for this situation. On reflection, Susan considered she had offered services to the family which she could not guarantee as she wanted to be accepted by them.

Social workers need to use communication skills in order to develop a rapport with service users and carers. However, having good communication skills will not guarantee that you will be able to form a relationship with the Gallagher family. Developing skills is only part of the required learning for social workers. As Ruch et al. (2010: 245) states, 'without the interest in and ability to work with human relationships, the social work task is diminished'. Relationships are influenced by socio-economic, political, cultural and agency contexts (Hennessey, 2001: 1). Social workers will also have individual views, personal values and assumptions about service users that will shape their relationships. An ability to respect and value diversity is an essential social work attribute, particularly when relating to people with different lifestyles and backgrounds, such as child-rearing practices, gender roles, sexual orientation, race and culture.

Relationships are at the core of social work. Forming and maintaining these relationships can be demanding, so practitioners need to develop emotional resilience and self-awareness. They need to 'recognize the impact of self in interacting with others' (PCF 1).

> The term 'self' is often used as a shorthand for a whole set of aspects of personality and identity including our personal beliefs and values, our anxieties and constructs – a combination of our rational and intuitive views on the way the world and other people operate and therefore on how we interact with the world and other people ... our 'self' is our primary tool of practice – it is the means through which we experience and conduct our practice, including the psychological and emotional demands which practice entails.
>
> (Ruch et al., 2010: 52)

The social work relationship forms the medium through which social work assessment, planning, intervention and review take place. Rogers (2012) believed that in order to develop a therapeutic relationship, three characteristics/conditions are needed: firstly 'empathy', which involves understanding how others feel and not making judgements about whether the feelings are right or wrong; secondly, 'warmth', which is accepting and caring for others and demonstrating 'unconditional positive regard'; and finally, being 'genuine', which means being ourselves, and not 'putting up a professional front or personal façade' (2012: 113).

There are also many different social work models and approaches which can be employed to develop relationships for specific purposes. These are discussed in more detail in Chapter 6 and include the psychosocial approach (Howe, 2002), play therapy (McMahon, 1992), solution-focused therapy (De Shazer and Dolan, 2007) and Rogers's person-centred approach (2012). The exchange model (Smale et al., 2000) of assessment recognises social worker expertise but regards service users as experts on themselves. This approach guides the communication process and empowers service users and carers. An important concept in communication theory is 'transferability' (Trevithick, 2012: 13). While recognising the central importance of relationships and the versatility of models and approaches, transferability requires social workers to adapt their knowledge and skills to different situations and apply their knowledge of human behaviour to individual service users.

Mastering Communication Skills: A Recipe

Initially students may be nervous about using their new skills and may follow their interview plan rigidly. However, as they gain experience and become more confident, they start to experiment and adapt skills and methods to different situations. The analogy of making a cake can be helpful. To bake a cake requires preparation, which usually starts with ensuring that you have the necessary ingredients and equipment. Likewise, for an interview, ingredients may include gathering information from the referral made by Jamie Gallagher's school and the database, which may give you more clues. Consider other professionals, such as the GP, who may know the family and be able to share information. You then need to write to the family to arrange a convenient appointment, that is, when the children are home from school.

The ingredients for the cake are now ready and you plan to follow the recipe. As with an interview, you need to think carefully about what methods you will employ to build a professional relationship with the family, based on respect, in order to gather information. Interviews are often time-limited, therefore considering your 'method' of communication and questioning is crucial. Think about using the core communication skills referred to earlier, of active listening, use of body language, demonstrating empathy, use of minimum encouragers such as nodding and smiling, questioning, clarifying, paraphrasing and summa (Egan, 2010). CHEFFLESH (see the Social History tool discussed later in this chapter) may also be another 'ingredient' to remind you of important areas for questioning – if the family are at risk of losing their tenancy through rent arrears, for example, this is likely to place them under stress; you need to know this. Your 'method' therefore is to bring all the ingredients together and blend them well. Forgetting to sieve the flour is likely to lead to a flat sponge, or for this analogy an unsuccessful interview, whereby you do not engage the family or glean important aspects of their daily lives.

The final stage, 'icing the cake', is perhaps how we end the interview – setting goals, summarising and discussing what happens next are as important as preparation and method. A wedding cake without icing could be viewed as unfinished and therefore not fit for purpose. As a novice you are likely to follow a 'recipe' exactly until you become more confident and 'expert'. Therefore substituting ingredients or forgetting to bring the assessment form to the interview is not necessarily a problem as you can use your expertise and initiative, such as by using a notebook to record the key assessment questions and answers.

Interviewing Skills and Tools

There are many different types of social work interviews such as an initial meeting, a home visit or a formal assessment. There may be a series of interviews over a period of time or there may only be the opportunity or need for one interview. This section will focus here on interviewing techniques, skills and tools that may help with planning and structuring interviews and taking social histories. Many social workers, students in particular, are often nervous about conducting interviews and benefit from engaging in simulated learning activities such as role-playing a first or potentially difficult home visit. In addition, students/social workers may find it helpful to have a written interview plan (Interviewing Tool 1.1).

Interviewing Tool 1.1: **Preparing an interview plan**

You may find it useful to prepare a written interview plan. You may want to write a checklist of things you need to remember. You might want to rehearse and write down what you will say and some generic open questions. You should aim to cover three stages of an interview: the beginning, middle and end.

1 Beginning

- Introduction – introduce your name and work title (being mindful of cultural competencies – shaking hands, eye contact, wearing shoes indoors, etc.).

- Confidentiality policy – you should explain what information might be shared with others.

- Gathering factual information – check the service user's/carer's name, DOB, address details and telephone number(s). Who else lives in the house? Closed questions are useful here to gather factual information.

2 Middle

- Purpose of the meeting – What is the purpose of the meeting? How much time have you got? Be clear about what you can and cannot do.

- Gathering information about the situation: 'their story' – utilise open questions, for example, 'So how can I help you today?' to start this process. As you progress, consider further questions such as 'tell me about your typical daily routine?'.

- Now write down three open questions below that you might use.

- Collate a social history.

3 End

- Endings – acknowledge the achievements and progress made by the service user or carer. What are you going to do in between now and your next meeting? Shake hands perhaps to formally end the meeting.

Having completed your interview plan, you can then proceed to think about how you would like to structure the interview. Whatever the purpose or setting, all interviews involve several stages (see Figure 1.1).

1 The first stage is to prepare for an interview. This involves undertaking research about the service user, agency policies and legislation; clarifying the purpose of the interview and context; and anticipating and 'tuning in to' how the

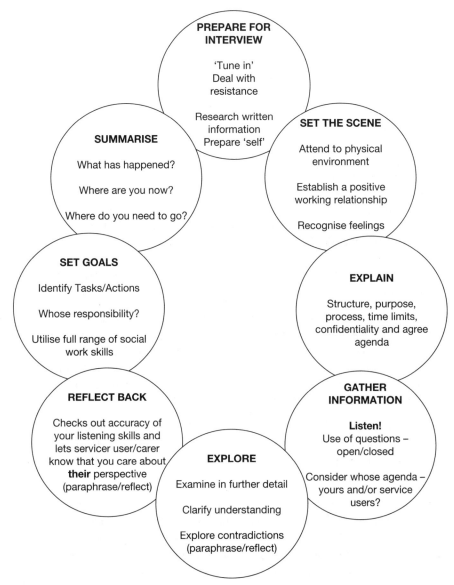

Figure 1.1 Interviewing tool: structuring an interview
Source: Trevithick (2012: 245).

service user might be feeling about the interview. The ability to engage in 'anticipatory empathy' (Kadushin and Kadushin, 2013: 129) and put ourselves in a service user's situation and understand their perspective is important. We can prepare for interviews by anticipating service users' feelings, such as anxiety, confusion, resistance or misconceptions about social workers.

'Mindfulness' involves being attuned to our instincts and gut feelings and allows social workers to 'perceive levels of distress and have a context in which they can assess its impact on them' (Rustin in Hennessey, 2001: 55).

Using the case example of the Gallagher family, we could prepare for the home visit anticipating that the family may be anxious about social work intervention and may fear that they will be judged. We could then identify strategies to address these concerns and reassure the family. Social workers need to begin interviews by establishing a shared understanding with the service user about the purpose, nature and process of the social work intervention. Agreeing on a shared agenda (Shulman, 2012) at the start of each interview or meeting enables all parties to have clear expectations and goals.

Davies (1994) describes an interview as a 'conversation with purpose'. This helps us focus on developing a rapport and getting to know the person. Effective social workers are able to put aside their own needs, and are able to focus solely on the service user and tune into their concerns (Shulman, 2012). Egan states that there should be four key stages in each intervention: exploration, understanding, action and evaluation (Egan, 2010).

2   The second stage of interviewing is to set the scene. This involves attending to the physical environment and establishing a positive relationship. If you have control over the interview venue, such as your office, you can plan the seating and provide toys for children. However, if you are making a home visit, you may have to deal with the unexpected, such as dogs barking, neighbours calling in and distractions like loud music and televisions.

3   The next stage is explaining the purpose of the interview. It is important to communicate about the structure, time limits and confidentiality of the interview, and agree on an agenda. For example, on a first home visit with the Gallagher family you could say:

> The purpose of today's meeting is to get to know you and explore the situation about Jamie's education. We have about an hour, and I would like to ask you some questions about the family and the children's education. I will respect your privacy and only share information on a need-to-know basis. I will be clear and honest with you about what I need to share and with whom.

4   Gathering information and questioning: Lishman (2009) and Koprowska (2010) summarise questioning as a key communication skill in order to gather information. Selecting the right questions in the correct sequence ensures that we establish the facts as well as explore the emotional context. A key skill with questioning is to be tactful and respectful, sprinkling questions naturally into conversation rather than asking multiple questions and interrogating people. When preparing to ask a sensitive question, it is helpful to begin by saying something like 'The next question is about your finances and you may find it intrusive – would it be ok to ask about this?'

Another way to gather information is through observation, paying attention to non-verbal communication, being sensitive to the atmosphere and mood and noticing any changes in behaviour.

5 Exploring further and clarifying: the exploration stage is crucial. Spending time at the beginning of an interview/intervention to really understand what is happening in the service user's life and to hear their story helps develop a rapport and a trusting relationship. Clarifying helps avoid making assumptions and errors and can save time later. For example, in the Gallagher case, you might make assumptions about the parents' culture and religion, based on personal experience or stereotypes of Irish people and the Catholic faith. Good practice would be to explore with Mr and Mrs Gallagher what their ethnicity and religion mean to them and their family. Questions such as 'How observant are you in regard to practising your religion?' and 'How would you identify yourself culturally?' may be posed. Careful use of brief pauses and therapeutic silence can be used to allow both the service user and interviewer space to reflect and gather their thoughts. Probing questions can be used to seek clarification and explore issues in depth.

6 Reflecting back what you have heard and observed is an important skill. The use of paraphrasing can check if you have listened attentively and will reassure the service user that you have understood what they have said. For example, Mrs Gallagher talks at length about her worries about money and drinking too much alcohol. The social worker paraphrases and says, 'it sounds like you are feeling stressed at the moment and that you are concerned about your rent arrears and your increased drinking'.

7 Setting goals: once you have established what the key concerns are, you can then proceed to agree on goals and an action plan. It is important to help service users identify priorities in order to deal with the most pressing issues first. For example, Mr and Mrs Gallagher may feel that they need help with their debts before they can address the other issues.

8 Summarising: Social workers often summarise throughout an interview as well as at the end. Agreeing on the main issues discussed and the goals set assists all parties to be clear and reassures service users that they have been heard and understood.

Taking a Social History: Tools for Assisting This

A social history is a holistic account of a person's circumstances which includes all the important factors, influences and changes that have contributed to their current situation. The process of communicating with service users and getting to know them allows social workers to explore each individual's personal story, enables the person to take charge of the information and decide on their priorities. In addition to gaining information from the service user, social workers can check case notes and reports and seek information from other professionals.

There are numerous tools that can be utilised here such as chronologies, eco maps and genograms which illustrate family history and relationships (SCIE, 2014). What do you think are the areas you may need to think about when completing a social history? Many agencies will have set formats, which will help guide you.

The acronym, CHEFFLESH, may help to remind you of key areas:

- Culture
  You may want to gain information about place of birth, languages spoken and the importance of culture to the individual and family.

- Health
  You will normally need to ask about physical and mental health. For instance, you may ask questions about any medical conditions, disabilities, medication, addictions, depression, anxiety and self-esteem. You may then explore if their health impacts on their general well-being, employment, finances, education or relationships.

- Education
  Questions can be posed to explore what education they have had, how education is experienced and valued and if there are any problems or specific learning needs.

- Family/Friends
  It is important to establish who the important people in service users' lives are and to explore the quality and stability of relationships. This process may reveal information about significant life events such as births, bereavements and separations. Once a trusting relationship is established, service users may feel able to share more sensitive information such as sexuality, intimate relationships, experiences of abuse and oppression.

- Finance
  Some service users will be reluctant to share details about their financial situations, so you may need to explain why you need this information. Understanding an individual's economic well-being can help identify any stresses such as debts, anxiety and instability.

- Leisure activities
  Getting to know the service user as a person, and not just someone with a problem, provides us with a holistic view of their interests, passions and talents. Gaining information about their leisure activities helps us identify their daily routine, lifestyle and strengths.

- Employment
  You may want to explore their employment history. Questions can be asked about hours of work, travelling time and impact on self and others.

- Spirituality
  Most agencies have standard questions about formal religion but it is also useful to explore what impact individual faith has on them and others. In addition to religions, service users may hold other values or belief systems.

- Housing
  Information can be sought to establish if the service user's home is appropriate for their needs. Is there easy access and sufficient space and amenities?

Self-preparation, Reflection and Feedback Skills

As part of continual learning and development, social work students and practitioners can gain from preparing themselves for new professional situations. They also need to consider how they use reflection to develop their self-awareness and ability to critically assess their strengths and areas for development. More on this is discussed in Chapter 8. Reflecting on experiences may involve seeking feedback, which together can assist with identifying gaps in knowledge or experience or particular training, education or consultation, mentoring or supervision needs, from a practice educator, manager or colleague.

You may find these preparatory and reflective activities helpful in relation to developing and improving communication and interviewing skills.

Learning Exercises 1.1: **To prepare yourself**

1 Practise your telephone skills by taking a referral over the phone – use the case study to practise with a colleague or friend.

2 Practise writing different kinds of letters, e.g. a letter to the family, arranging a home or an office visit, feeding back on an eligibility assessment for services (whether they qualify or not).

3 Role-play a home visit: in front of a mirror, practise your introduction, questions and ending, as well as monitoring your facial expressions. You need to feel confident and relaxed. Anxiety may cause you to look stern, so make sure you smile on occasion.

4 Role-play a network meeting – colleagues, family or friends to practise public speaking and delivering information.

5 Role-play a review meeting – colleagues, family or friends to practise public speaking, delivering information and ensuring you work inclusively with the service user or carer.

Reflective Exercise 1.2: **Using critical reflection skills when practising interviews**

Are you aware of your strengths and weaknesses in communicating with service users? Do you know how service users see you?

It is good practice to regularly seek feedback from service users and carers, colleagues, practice educators and managers about our practice. It is important to be open and responsive to feedback and to reflect on our skills, identifying both what we do well and what we need to improve.

A useful learning exercise is to record yourself using audio and visual technology, such as a dictaphone, mobile phone or camcorder. Do you sound different to how you imagined? How is your body language? Do you have a default facial expression? Have you any distracting habits such as fidgeting, interrupting, clicking your pen or repeating the same words?

In order to become more reflexive as practitioners, we need to increase our self-awareness and extend our knowledge of our 'blind spots' and gain insight into how others regard us (Johari Window in Luft and Ingham, 1955).

Peer and Service User and Carer Feedback

Feedback is a useful tool when learning new skills. When role-playing and practising communication, students and colleagues can give each other feedback on their skills. In addition, feedback is provided to students on placement by practice educators and to qualified social workers by their line managers. It is important to discuss ground rules about feedback and make a written agreement about how you want to do this. Feedback should be constructive, objective and specific. People often remember the negative comments they receive and somehow block off the positive feedback, so we recommend beginning and ending feedback with positive comments. One model of feedback is called a 'feedback sandwich', that is, two pieces of positive feedback are wrapped around any negative comments or suggestions for improvement. Pendleton's rules are also important (Moss, 2008: 111) for oral feedback on communication skills. Pendleton's model begins with student self-evaluation and identifying what went well. Once the strengths have been identified, then a discussion is had about what could have been done differently. The other students and the tutors then comment on strengths and areas for improvement.

Students at university may have the opportunity for live feedback on their communication skills in Practice Learning Suites/Skills Labs, where students are recorded while practising their skills and then watch themselves back on video screen. They may also receive feedback from peers, tutors, service users and carers, and practice educators. This feedback helps students to reflect and supports the development of self-awareness. It also provides an opportunity to learn to value peer review and peer support.

The form in Table 1.1 provides a useful structure when soliciting comments/feedback from others. This can be completed by a practice educator, academic tutor, manager/supervisor, colleague or fellow student, and/or adapted for service user/carer feedback.

Gaining feedback from service users and carers in both learning and practice arenas is vital to improve individual and practice skills. Evaluation and feedback may be part of an agency's systems, but it is also good practice to seek opportunities to find ways of hearing their views on your individual practice.

Table 1.1 Sample feedback form: communication skills

Did the interviewer use minimal encouragers?	Yes/No
What was good about the interviewer's non-verbal skills?	
What non-verbal skills would have improved the interview?	
Did the interviewer use open questions?	Yes/No Give an example
Did the interviewer use paraphrasing or reflection?	Yes/No Give an example
Did the interviewer clarify issues effectively?	Yes/No Give an example
Did the interviewer effectively?	
How was the ending managed?	
Anything else you would like to tell your colleague about the interview?	

Conclusion

Effective communication skills prepare a professional social worker for specific tasks such as interviewing, but it is also essential in other professional contexts, such as multidisciplinary meetings and collaboration. While these skills are a requirement of first-level qualifying education, they need to be continually reviewed and refreshed by social work practitioners in order to be able to transfer them to each unique service user situation and deal with new challenges in complex and changing professional contexts.

Progress check

As part of meeting the Professional Capabilities Framework (PCF) and the Health and Care Professions Council (HCPC)'s Standards of Proficiency (HCPC 2012b), you will need to continually develop your communication skills, whether you are a student, newly qualified social worker or experienced practitioner. This chapter focuses on specific communication and interviewing skills, micro skills and techniques and tools that will enable social workers to 'enable effective relationships' and be 'effective communicators' (PCF 7 Intervention & Skills) and to continue to meet HCPC Standards 1, 3, 7, 8 and 9.

Students need to show development prior to placement, between placements and by the end of the last placement, and at this juncture, communication and interviewing skills will be particularly rigorously assessed, taking special note of feedback from service users and carers. A key issue, particularly for students and newly qualified social workers, is learning from experience and feedback; and some suggestions and tools made in this chapter for learning and reflection exercises and for gaining feedback from others may assist with PCF 7 in the evaluation 'of their own practice'. Basic skills, such as active listening, questioning, clarifying, paraphrasing and summarising, are also relevant to skills applied to multi-professional communication and how they are seen in collaborative work with other professionals (PCF 8).

Links to the professionalism domain (PCF 1) identify also how social workers can continue to 'demonstrate professional commitment by taking responsibility for their conduct, practice and learning, with support through supervision', particularly in relation to their communication and interviewing skills, and the maintenance of social work values (HCPC 2012a) and ethical practice (PCF 2).

Newly qualified practitioners will find that their reflection on skills learnt on their qualifying courses will enable them to show how they have developed and improved their confidence and expertise, when meeting the Assessed and Supported Year in Employment (ASYE) requirements (The College of Social Work 2014). They, and all qualified social workers, could use reflection on communication skills as part of their portfolio for HCPC's re-registration/CPD requirements.

Managing communication with service users and carers in different roles in different settings (working in many and varied organisations, PCF 7) can put extra challenges and complexity into how social workers maintain their abilities to be authoritative and assertive, while retaining compassion and empathy. This chapter suggests ways of using role-play, consultation, mentoring and supervision to develop social worker awareness of how they and their communication are perceived by others, and the need to 'recognize the impact of self in interacting with others' (PCF 1), which students need to demonstrate by the point of assessment of readiness for direct practice (prior to first placement).

Skillfully communicating with service users from different cultures, faiths and sexual orientations and managing conflict and dealing with resistance and hostility are all areas for advancement within professional practice, taking into account the high degree of specialism within current social work roles, and the increasing recognition of the need for emotional resilience.

Chapter Summary

The aim of this chapter is to enable social work students and new practitioners to identify and improve their communication skills in social work practice. It refers to a range of literature and identifies core principles, skills and knowledge for effective communication, as well as factors affecting communication skills and the context in which they are exercised. In addition to making links to communication as part of professionalism, specific guidance, resources and strategies are provided on communication and interviewing micro skills, relationship building, planning and structuring interviews with service users and carers and taking social histories. A case study provides an example for practice and reflection on interviewing. The chapter focuses on communicating with service users and carers although many of the skills can be transferred to relating to all people and settings such as inter-professional working.

Examples of activities to support the development of communication and interviewing skills are provided, including exercises for self-preparation, reflection on skills and receiving feedback from peers, practice educators, service users and carers and other professionals.

Further Reading

- Egan, G. (2010) *The Skilled Helper: A Problem Management and Opportunity Development Approach*, 9th edition. CA: Brookes/Cole.
- Koprowska, J. (2010) *Communication and Interpersonal Skills in Social Work*, 3rd edition. Exeter: Learning Matters.
- Social Care Institute for Excellence (SCIE) e-learning resources, available at http://www.scie.org.uk/publications/elearning/communicationskills/index.asp.
- Social Care TV, available at http://www.scie.org.uk/socialcaretv/index.asp.
- Trevithick, P. (2012) *Social Work Skills and Knowledge*. Berkshire: McGraw Hill: Open University Press.

References

Croisdale-Appleby, D. (2014) Re-visioning Social Work Education, an Independent Review, available at https://www.gov.uk/government/uploads/system/uploads/attachment_data/file/285788/DCA_Accessible.pdf.
Davies, M. (1994) *The Essential Social Worker*, 3rd edition. Aldershot: Ashgate.
De Shazer, S. and Dolan, Y. (2007) *More than Miracles: The State of the Art of Solution-focused Brief Therapy*. New York: Haworth Press.
Doel, M. and Shardlow, S. (2005) *Modern Social Work Practice*. Aldershot: Ashgate.

Egan, G. (2010) *The Skilled Helper: A Problem Management and Opportunity Development Approach,* 9th edition. CA: Brookes/Cole.

HCPC (2012a) Standards of Proficiency, available at http://www.hcpcuk.org/publications/standards/index.asp?id=569

HCPC (2012b) Guidance on Conduct & Ethics for Students, available at http://www.hpc-uk.org/publications/brochures/index.asp?id=219

Healy, K. and Meagher, G. (2004) The Re-professionalisation of Social Work: Collaborative Approaches for Achieving Professional Recognition, *British Journal of Social Work,* 34 (2): 243–260.

Hennessey, R. (2001) *Relationship Skills in Social Work.* London: Sage.

Howe, D. (2002) Psychosocial Work In: Social Work: themes, issues and critical debates.

Koprowska, J. (2010) *Communication and Interpersonal Skills in Social Work,* 3rd edition. Exeter: Learning Matters.

Lishman, J. (2009) *Communication and Social Work,* 2nd edition. Basingstoke: Palgrave MacMillan.

Luft, J. and Ingham, H. (1955) *The Johari Window, A Graphic Model of Interpersonal Awareness.* Los Angeles: UCLA.

Macmillan Kadushin, A. and Kadushin, G. (2013) *The Social Work Interview,* 5th edition. New York: Columbia University Press.

McMahon, L. (1992) *The Handbook of Play Therapy.* London: Routledge.

Moss, B. (2008) *Communication Skills for Health and Social Care.* London: Sage.

Munro, E. (2011) *The Munro Review of Child Protection: A Child-centred System.* Department for Education: The Stationery Office Limited

Phillips, A. (2013) *Developing Assertiveness Skills for Health and Social Care Professionals.* Milton Keynes: Radcliffe Publishing.

Rogers, C. (2012) *Client Centred Therapy,* New edition. London: Constable and Robinson.

Ruch, G., Turney, D. and Ward, A. (2010) *Relationship-Based Social Work.* London: Jessica Kingsley Publications.

SCIE e-learning resource on communication skills (2014) (http://www.scie.org.uk/assets/elearning/communicationskills/cs04/resource/html/object4/object4_7.htm#slide01)

Shulman, L. (2012) *The Skills of Helping Individuals, Families, Groups and Communities,* 7th edition. Itasca, IL: F.E. Peacock.

Smale, G. and Tuson, G., with Biehal, N. and Statham, D. (2000) *Social Work and Social Problems.* Basingstoke: Macmillan.

The College of Social Work (2014) Assessed and supported year in employment, available at http://www.skillsforcare.org.uk/Social-work/Assessed-and-Supported-Year-in-Employment/The-Assessed-and-Supported-Year-in-Employment-(ASYE).aspx

Trevithick, P. (2012) *Social Work Skills and Knowledge: A Practice Handbook.* 3rd edition, Milton Keynes: Open University Press.

2

WRITING SKILLS FOR SOCIAL WORKERS

Ray Jones

Introduction

This chapter focuses on why writing well is a required competence for social workers. Consideration is given to the purposes for which a social worker might write, what helps to write well and the tools and techniques which promote good writing. The range of writing required by social workers is noted, with sections on recording, report writing, letters and, increasingly important, emails, texts and social media. These latter forms of communication are increasingly being used in keeping in touch with young people, but they also have risks if it is forgotten that they should still be embedded within the professional relationship.

In essence, whilst much attention is often given to the importance of, and competence required in, face-to-face exchanges, interviewing and verbal (and non-verbal) communications, less attention may have been given to the ability to write well, as communication, as a record and to assist reflection and clarification. This chapter seeks to address each of these issues.

It is not difficult to see that badly written scripts, as noted below, cause confusion and may create misunderstandings, and when the writing is very poor, it is likely that all that is written will not be read as it is too time-consuming and taxing. So, written skills are important for social workers.

The Range and Reach of Writing Required by Social Workers

Having writings skills is not about always writing in the same style. We all show preferences and quirks within our writing, as is considered in the Reflective Exercise 2.1 below.

Reflective Exercise 2.1

Some people are heavy users of alliteration, using words in relation to each other which start with the same letter and sound. Some are prone to rather generously sprinkle exclamation marks for emphasis.

What are the personal characteristics of your writing style? List them. Then ask someone else to look at a couple of pieces you have written and to comment on anything they have spotted about your style. Think about whether these personal characteristics are acceptable and likely to be agreeable to others or whether they are likely to be a hindrance and annoyance.

But it is important to have flexible writing styles as writing is for different purposes. It would not be exceptional, for example, for a social worker to arrive in their office in the morning and to read and respond to emails from others in the organisation, to dictate or type a letter to a client arranging to visit later in the week, to prepare a review report about a family for a meeting involving other agencies and to write up the previous day's visits. The social worker might also be leading a project or activity and may need to write a bid to justify its funding or a newsletter to inform a dispersed and disparate readership about what is happening. Each of these activities has its own requirements in terms of how it is being written. Some of these differing requirements will be explored in more detail below, but here is a list of possible considerations on intended purposes to take into account when thinking about writing style (adapted from Hopkins, 1998a: 10):

- To inform [tell]
- To find out [ask]
- To persuade [convince]
- To enforce [demand and require]
- To record [organise and capture]

Each of these intended purposes will require that the writer is clear about what they are seeking to achieve and the style of writing will vary. For example, to enforce is likely to require directness, explicit clarity and more formality, whereas to persuade may need to capture the reader's commitment and have more explanation. Healy and Mulholland (2009) argue for a 'contextual approach' to writing with the elements of 'institutional context' (the agency, but also the context of legislation and policy), 'professional purpose' (what is the intention that the writing should achieve) and 'audience' (who are the intended readers that will read what is written). Much of what follows in this chapter emphasise the above context.

But, first, if there is any doubt about the requirement to write well, consider Case Study 2.1 below.

Case Study 2.1: **Writing badly**

So, what might it be like if a social worker wrote badly? What if the social worker wrote 'When i visited mr's Smith it was a mess'. There are two immediate problems here beyond the misuse, in this instance underuse, of capital letters. First, who was visited, Mr or Mrs Smith? Second, what was a mess? Was it the visit and had the social worker possibly not prepared for it well? Or it was the house which was visited which was a mess? Anyone reading this would have to guess what meaning should be attached to the short, badly written, sentence.

It hardly inspires confidence that here is a social worker who thinks clearly, has a positive impact by communicating well and who would have credibility with others. It should be an embarrassment for the social worker and would be for the agency.

When reflecting on badly written scripts, it is not difficult to see the confusion they may create and the misunderstandings which might occur, and when the writing is very poor, it is likely that all that is written will not be read as it is too time-consuming and taxing. So, written skills are important for social workers.

Considering the context of any written communication is important in deciding how best to write. *Purpose* is one of the determinants of writing style. The second would be the *readership*. Writing a letter to a child requires a consideration of what is likely to be understandable within that stage of a child's linguistic and comprehension ability. Writing a report to be read by a high court judge may reasonably assume greater ability and capacity. But the report to the judge will also be read by, and needs to be understandable to, others, including parents and indeed possibly older children. The differences in comprehension ability are why official reports may have easy-to-read versions as well as the original full version. It is often found that the easy-to-read versions of reports are (deliberately) much clearer and easier to assimilate than the original. Why? Because as Hopkins has noted for himself 'I realised I was writing to impress and not writing to inform' (Hopkins, 1998b: 2). What, however, is usually impressive is good writing to inform. Writing to impress with lots of jargon – or as in legal documents archaic expressions and a lack of punctuation – is likely to be seen as a sign of arrogance, possibly insecurity and probably incompetence. So KISS – keep it simple stupid!

Third, in addition to purpose and audience, there is *context*. Correspond-ence between family and friends may allow, indeed benefit from, a familiarity and informality. Writing from a formal agency role, where the role is not primarily about friendship but about the professional task, requires some distance to be kept. But this does not mean a retreat into officialese and bureaucracy– or management-speak. It means using everyday words but without colloquial, cultural and generational-specific written communica-tion and conversation which is acceptable between friends and is indeed indicative of friendship and informality. This is not just an issue for social workers and their written communication. How to engage and be empa-thetic with others whilst appropriately maintaining a professional relation-ship with its inherent boundaries (and power) always requires reflection and maintenance.

The Tools and Techniques of Writing

All writers have several tools at hand. First there are words. These are joined in sentences and these in turn are brought together and also broken up into para-graphs, which are then spread across pages. This might all seem rather obvious and basic. But choosing which words to use, spelling them correctly, linking them together into sentences and then deciding on a structure for the text can at each stage be rather more challenging.

There are five 'S's at play here:

- Selection

- Spelling

- Sentences

- Structure

- Shape

Selecting the words is assisted by having a larger vocabulary. This in turn is likely to result from being an avid reader as well as a writer. But even when having a large vocabulary from which to choose, how is it decided which words to use? Again, wherever possible KISS – keep it simple stupid. For example, something is 'contested' means there is disagreement about it, but 'contested' which means 'disputed' is not a term used by most people, albeit more frequently used in academic papers.

And then there are terms which come into fashion but have the potential to confuse rather than clarify. For example, a plan is now a 'road map', but really there are no roads and there is no map; it is just a plan. If the intention is to communicate and clarify, avoid jargon and complexity. Keep it straight and simple.

Also work hard on getting spellings accurate, as misspellings not only undermine credibility but can also lead to misunderstandings, as noted in Case Study 2.2.

Case Study 2.2: **Carelessness and confusion**

Be careful to avoid confusion. It is not a good idea to write 'He told me about his cash find' if what was meant was 'he told me about his cash fine'. Only one letter is different: in the first more money; in the second less money. And if the punctuation is changed, so is the meaning – 'He told me about his cash, fine' – so it was ok that he told me about his money. Or how about 'she was concerned about her sight' when what she was really concerned about was her new location, her site. Context may help spot errors and mistakes but carelessness can be recklessness. Carelessness costs in written communications.

Having a dictionary and thesaurus at hand, and using them, is a good habit. So is proof checking the draft before finalising it. Be careful though with proof reading. It is not just about reading back through the text, as what is read is often what was intended rather than what has been written. Proof reading requires a deliberate activity of consciously looking at what is on the page or screen. Use, but also be careful, of spell checkers and predictive text – software spell checkers often offer and introduce Americanised spellings, and predictive text corrections can be bizarre.

Bringing words together into *sentences* is another challenge and one with more complexity requiring an understanding of punctuation and the rules of grammar. Lynn Truss (2003) created a bestselling book about it. Is her book title really about pandas and dining ('eats shoots and leaves') or about an angry and ungrateful dinner guest ('eats, shoots and leaves')? And here is a real-life example from a book about recording in social work – a subheading reads 'Essential but pointless: attitudes to recording' (O'Rourke, 2010). This says what the author meant, that social workers often saw recording as pointless but it was still essential to do it. But leave out the colon and it reads 'Essential but pointless attitudes to recording' where the meaning is now that the attitudes are pointless.

There are common mistakes to be seen over and over again in the writings of social workers and of others. May be it is seen as a sign of cleverness to add punctuation unnecessarily and indeed erroneously. When writing about a gathering of GPs, there seems to be widely shared urge to write GP's. The first, GPs, is about more than one GP. The second is about something belonging to a GP. Two books by Hopkins (1998a, 1998b) are useful, fun to read and aids to improve spellings and grammar.

Moving beyond spellings and sentences, there is the shape and structure of what is written. And the same rule applies. KISS – keep it simple stupid. The task when writing is not only to present accurately what it is intended to record or communicate but also to help the future reader, who might indeed be the writer themselves sometime in future, to recognise and retrieve the information within the written script. This is made easier if the information is presented in blocks which structure the reader's attention.

But first, back to sentences. Information in shorter sentences is easier to assimilate than lots of information in a longer sentence with no breaks. Longer sentences often require re-reading as too much is being communicated to be captured in one reading.

The same is true of paragraphs. Shorter paragraphs, containing what is relevant about one point or one argument, allow the reader to identify this as a block of information which has coherence and relevance and to be understood and remembered as such by the reader. Long, often rambling, paragraphs, like long sentences, add complexity and lead to potential confusion or lack of comprehension. Just think, for example, how much more difficult it would be to spot the points just made if the three paragraphs above were merged into a much longer single paragraph.

So thinking about the *shape of paragraphs* is important. It is also important to think about the overall *structure* of what is being written. Remember the task is to record so that information is easy to retrieve or to communicate with others who can understand what is being said and shared. Simple and short sentences and paragraphs are the building blocks but the whole edifice – the total text – needs to have a unity and to be recognisable.

This is where breaking up the texts with sign posts and pause spaces can be helpful. Chapters in a longer formal report assist the reader to understand and to search for where particular issues or information may be located. Headings and subheadings in a file record or a court or other report again helps the reader to navigate through the argument and information in the text and to spot changes in content and focus.

But text can be broken up and divided in other ways, especially when the intention is to draw attention to particular parts of the text. **Type-face** and **size** might be changed to emphasise a particular issue – bold and a bigger **type-face** as used in this sentence; italic as in previous parts of this chapter. Boxing text or using bullet points, as in this chapter, also helps to highlight and draw attention to particular text and themes. But do NOT *overdo* it or it all becomes **too complex**. The aim is to be helpful to the reader as they structure their reading of the text but do not make it messy, complicated and confusing.

Here are some bullet points as a reminder of key points above about tools and techniques to be kept in mind when writing (and alliteration, using a sequence or words starting with the same letter, can also be helpful to readers in remembering points):

- Spelling and semantics [the meaning of words]
- Sentences
- Shape
- Structure

And here is another bullet point list to draw attention to what to do when the written text has been first drafted, and do see it as first draft. Always, even when in a rush, do check what has been written and follow through on the four 'R's below:

- Read
- Reflect
- Review
- Revise

The most difficult task can be DISCARDING and DESTROYING what is not necessary and what is not pertinent. It sometimes is difficult to take out what has some value and point, but which really is superfluous to what should be recorded or communicated. Whilst writing, and in the midst of a stream of thought, it is easy to get a little carried away, to become unfocused and to go off on a tangent. Again, for the reader, this adds unnecessary complexity, so in addition to KISS – keep it simple stupid, do STICK TO THE KNITTING and stay focused on what is necessary and essential.

Two reflections: First, repetition sometimes helps to drive points home – by now the underlying message of KISS should be recognised and remembered as it has been repeated several times in this chapter. Second, the KISS and 'stick to the knitting' messages were driven home in a management book of the 1980s which attracted considerable attention and interest at the time (Peters and Waterman, 1982), so there are messages here which do not only relate to writing but also to how to structure so much of what needs to be done in social work and elsewhere – seek to keep it simple and focused.

Just in case there is any confusion, thinking about shape and structure when writing is not only a task when reviewing and revising at the end of the process. It is one of the first issues to be considered, after having given thought to what is to be recorded or communicated, why and with what intended impact and for which potential readership.

It may also be helpful to prepare a guide to assist the reader to know what is ahead and how it is structured. So here is a note about what is to follow:

Writing for different purposes:

- Case recording

- Letters

- Reports to others

Writing in different media:

- Paper

- Computer-based recording

- Emails

- Texting

- Social media

Summary and reflections:

- Remembering and reinforcing the main points

- Linking again to the PCF and SoP.

So, the shape and outline content of what is now to be written (and read) is known. This is helpful not only for the writer in getting it written but also for the reader in recognising and indeed later retrieving what is in the text. It is the same when giving or listening to a lecture. It is helpful to understand what is to come in terms of content, structure and sequence as a means of recognising how it all links and fits together while still having bite-size chunks which can be remembered.

Progress Check

Being able to communicate and being able to record are stated as central to the role of social workers. For example:

- Standard of Proficiency (SoP) 8 (*Be able to communicate effectively*) is related to Professional Capabilities Framework (PCF) 7 (*Intervention and skills*), which includes skills in communication (7.1) and influence and persuasion (7.2).

▶

- SoP 10 (*Be able to maintain records appropriately*) relates to PCF 7.8 (*Meet legislative and agency responsibilities and requirements*).

Possibly, less obviously, writing skills may also be seen as required by SoP 4 (*Be able to practice as an autonomous professional, exercising their own professional judgement*). In particular, SoP 4.4 (*Be able to make informed judgements on complex issues using the information available*) is assisted by being able to record information so that it can be critically appraised by the social workers (SoP11.1) and in supervision (SoP 11.2). In essence, writing to communicate and to record is important, but writing to aid thinking and reflection is also an additional opportunity.

Writing for Different Purposes

Recording

Recording is rarely the most popular activity for social workers. It may be seen as a distraction from the real work of social workers and to divert activity away from contact with service users. But, may be surprisingly, the amount of social workers' direct service user contact time has changed little over the years (see summary in Jones et al., 2013). A recent study reported in the same paper by different professionals working in health and social care teams found that while community nurses spent 32% of their time in direct contact with patients, this was less than 20% for social workers (but also for occupational therapists).

So, what are the social workers doing when not in direct contact with service users? The 2012 study found that they spend 29% of their time on recording and report writing (19% for community nurses). Therefore, here is another reason why writing skills for social workers are important. If so much time is spent on writing, it is a good idea to at least do it well.

So, why is so much (too much?) time spent on recording? Why should one spend time on recording at all? This is explored in the Reflective Exercise 2.2

Reflective Exercise 2.2: **Place in rank order your views of why it is important to record**

- Accountability – for work undertaken and decisions made.
- Insurance – you can show and demonstrate what you have done and why you have done it.

- Fulfilling statutory requirements.

- Generating performance data and information.

- Information sharing – someone else can take informed action when you are not available.

- Reflection – you can consider with your supervisor or others what is happening and what sense to make of it.

- Structuring thinking – the process of recording is helpful in clarifying your own thoughts.

- Any other views you may have not listed above.

Comments from others about recording are noted below. Note how the requirement, process and content has changed over time, especially with what has been seen as the increased focus on managerial oversight and control and recoding to generate performance information:

> Social work is a complex, ambiguous and often uncertain business and audit is increasingly being used to hold individual practitioners and their agencies to account.
>
> (O'Rourke, 2010: 30)

> There is the professional aim of producing timely and sufficiently detailed recording so that, for example, someone else can continue the work if the allocated social workers is ill. But, arguably, the more significant drivers behind the development of ICS [the Integrated Children's System database] are managerial and supervisory. By making social workers record their visits to looked-after children on a central database it is easy to monitor their work and to send reminders if they are in danger of not meeting the minimum frequency for statutory visits.
>
> (Hill and Shaw, 2011: 29)

But what has possibly received less attention and recognition is how recording may be a process which facilitates and clarifies assessments, appraising options and assisting with planning future actions. It ought to be a part of the process of critical analysis. Just the process of deciding what to write and how to set out text requires structured thinking. It also requires reflection on what to include and what to exclude. The records then are available to feed the discussion in supervision.

Records are also of importance in providing information and a briefing for others who may become involved with a service user when the social worker is not available. This is where having well-structured records should help colleagues to see what has happened in the past, what is the most recent assessment and action plan, and to match the response to the service user with the assessment and plan. Indeed, it may be helpful to see case recording in four parts:

- The running record of information and action.

- Regular summaries with the frequency determined by the amount of activity and also by the rate and pace of change.

- Assessments and reviews which are updated at regular intervals or when there is significant change.

- Plans which are regularly updated.

Giving a narrative and telling a story through recording are important as these both give an account of information and actions over time and also joins them up so that they have meaning. But telling the story is not about story-telling as in writing fiction. The narrative needs to be firmly grounded in reality and evidence, and it is often helpful and sensible to make it clear what is factual and what may be opinion or supposition.

Creating and telling the story is not, however, helped by the fragmentation and pre-defined categorisation generated by computerised recording where information has to be recorded and shaped within pre-determined formats (see Seymour and Seymour, 2011). This may generate data such as how many children aged zero to four have child protection plans, how many older people are receiving 10+ hours of home care a week or how long is the time interval between referral and first contact with a service user, all of which may be necessary for nationally or locally determined performance indicator reports. It will allow performance comparisons between and within agencies and over time. This is important, and it is one of the levers central government, in particular, has used to drive performance improvement. But for individual assessments and case planning, it may be a hindrance as it fragments information into data and undermines the telling and seeing of the overall picture. This tension between generating data to feed the performance reporting agenda and using recording to tell and see the story remains unresolved in many information systems:

> There is evidence that the evaluation of ICS [the Integrated Children's System database] to show that social workers and their managers have concerns about the tendency of ICS exemplars to break up 'the story' in such a way as to make it difficult to understand the whole picture.
>
> (Hill and Shaw op cit.: 82)

> The electronic recording and retrieving system does not effectively support staff in undertaking their work ... The combination of no single record for a child and not all

files having chronologies makes it difficult to ensure that all historical information is taken into account in assessment and decision-making.

(Ofsted, 2010: 173)

But case records have two other important functions. First, when service users have shared and open-access to records, it promotes measured statements and judgements within the records. It also may assist in promoting the work with service users as a shared enterprise with the user, and it provides an opportunity to make issues and views explicit and to give them emphasis.

Case records are also a part of responsibility sharing within the agency. They move on from the contact between service users and workers being only an unseen, and potentially secret, activity. They should make the contact known to others and should be more transparent. And a further extension of this theme is that they provide a degree of insurance for the worker (and service user) as they give a relatively contemporary account of what has happened which can be referred to if there should be future concerns. This will never be a water-tight insurance policy as it can always be challenged in terms of truthfulness. It is in part why professional regulators such as the Health and Care Professions Council (HCPC) for social workers take very seriously the falsifying of records as this undermines the credibility of the recording process as well as demonstrating the lack of integrity of the writer of the records.

By way of concluding this section on recording, and to reinforce the points above, here is a quote which echoes the earlier statement about the importance of recording and that it is a part of the social work task and not a distraction from the real work:

If all these points [about the reasons for case recording] elevate the case record to a position of great importance in daily social work practice, then this is what we intend. Case records as important social actions in casework are worth as much time as you can give them.

(Healy and Mulholland, op. cit.: 72)

Report Writing

In addition to case recording, social workers write reports for a range of purposes. They might, as with reports to case conferences or to support a referral to other workers or agencies, be about *information sharing*. Indeed all reports will at least in part be about providing information. But some reports will also be about trying to *persuade and influence* others, such as reports advocating on behalf of service users to housing or benefits agencies. And some reports will be about providing *professional judgements and advice* to assist others in their decision-making, as with reports to courts.

The comments earlier in this chapter about writing well can now be seen to be especially important. Reports need to have clarity, and report writers need to write well to have credibility, if they are to be useful to others and to have influence and impact. As with case recording, spending time on report writing in non-contact client time is not a distraction from the real work of social workers. It is a part of the real day job. Direct contact and work with service users is important, but so usually is informing, influencing and having impact on others.

With report writing, how the text is structured is particularly important. The structure needs to help the reader to see how the information provided, or the argument being made, breaks down into its different elements. This aids the reader's understanding and comprehension. If trying to persuade the reader, the structure of the text with headings, subheadings and paragraphs, and maybe with bullet point lists and highlighting for emphasis, takes the reader through the milestones of a thought-journey which hopefully might end at the intended destination of the reader agreeing with the writer and accepting the writer's request or recommendation.

In report writing, especially for reports that are intended to inform and influence decision-making and which may be contested and challenged, such as court reports, it is important to explicitly differentiate between fact, analysis and opinion, and to show how the opinion is evidence-informed, as noted below:

> Professional opinions expressed in a report should always be based on analysis of material contained on that report. Everyone who reads it should be clear on what facts your opinion is based, to what extent you have personal knowledge of those facts and the source of any facts of which you do not have personal knowledge, such as case records made before you took over the case.
>
> (Seymour and Seymour, op. cit.: 109)

As reports can take on a life of their own well beyond their immediate purpose and even beyond the involvement of the report writer, it is important that they are measured and modest in what they contain. They become a part of the historic record and will have a life lasting well beyond the time at which they were written, and as such they should be dated and the author named.

Again, KISS – keep it simple stupid, and as Lishman has noted about court reports:

> It needs to be written in clear, straightforward language. It should avoid professional jargon. The use of such phrases as 'structural factors', 'deviant sub-culture' or 'material deprivation' alienate the non-social work reader.
>
> (Lishman, 2009: 56)

As commented upon above, the intention is to inform and influence and not to impress, albeit a well-structured, well-written and easy-to-read report will impress and be authoritative.

Letters

Reflecting on letters sent through the post, or delivered by hand, may seem a little archaic. After all, surely letters have largely been replaced by emails (memos certainly have largely become defunct). But letters have a particular value and function, even when delivered by email.

First, not everyone has email or computer access and still receives their written correspondence through the letterbox. Even when there is the option of email, a letter can, depending on how it is written, portray greater formality or, indeed, greater personalization (as in a letter of condolence). And this is of importance. When writing a letter, consideration needs to be given to how to position and present oneself in relation to the reader as well as what information is to be conveyed in the letter. A letter can be very informal or formal, personal or official, whereas reports are always formal, and emails tend to be less formal, often starting 'Hi there' rather than 'Dear'.

In letter writing, attention should be given to the degree of formality to be used, and this starts with the initial term of address to the recipient and reader and ends with how the letter writer chooses to describe themselves. For example, when writing to a service user who is well known to the letter writer, it may be acceptable to address the letter to 'Dear Jane', but a letter arranging an initial meeting will more appropriately be addressed to 'Dear Ms Johnson'. And signing a letter as 'Mary Brown' or 'Mrs Mary Brown' with the signature as 'Mary', 'Mary Brown' or 'M. Brown' is likely to depend on type and extent of relationship with the letter recipient. It may also be influenced by the age of the recipient with letters to children less formal and letters to adults possibly more formally addressed. But even when less formal, it is still important to remain professional:

> All letters have to show professionalism in the way the [letter] format is used, for example the correct cultural procedures, good layout with a good choice of font and appropriate spacing, as well as by the letter's logically developed content and a language free from slang and jargon.
>
> (Healy and Mulholland, op. cit.: 59)

Emails, Texts and Social Media

This is the time to be very careful and cautious. The quicker it is possible to write, send and receive, and the wider the audience which can be achieved, should lead the writer to be very deliberate and decisive about what is written. It is too late once an email or text has been sent, or once it has been lodged on a social media site, to want to reclaim and revise what has been written. It is already out of control.

The same rules should apply to emails as to any other writing with a professional purpose. They should be well structured and well written. Spelling and punctuation should be correct and although emails and texts amongst friends and family may have an informality, the requirements of a professional presentation and style still hold when using email and texts to communicate when in a professional role. The message still needs to be professionally structured and styled even if the medium is often used for non-professional purposes in social exchanges.

Particular care should be taken by social workers and other professionals when using social media, even when it is being used outside of the professional role. Once available to a wide readership, and even if not intended by its author, it gives a picture – sometimes in words and sometimes graphically and visually – to a wider audience and public. This crossing and merging of the private and public, the personal and the professional, means that Facebook and LinkedIn, with their filing of party and family photos, and of opinion and accounts of holidays and histrionics, may be available not only to friends and families but to other professionals, managers, the press and the public at large, including service users.

First, maybe the informality of social media is more likely to encourage opinionated, unguarded and personalised comment. Second, when making these comments, free and extensive access to the comments means that it will not take long for others to be alerted to the comments. And third, it is too late after the comment has been published in the Twitter-sphere to wish instead that it had been consigned to a waste-paper bin, which was always an option when reading the first draft of a letter on paper. It is sensible, therefore, to be wary and wise about the use and misuse of social media, and guidance has been provided for social workers (BASW, 2012).

Conclusion

Hopefully this chapter has reinforced the statements in the PCF and SoP about being skilled in writing is one of the competencies required of social workers. It has relevance if social workers are to perform well in their roles of informing and influencing others and also in being reflective themselves. Being a skilled writer is not, however, about seeking to impress. A recurrent theme throughout this chapter has been to KISS – keep it simple stupid. Communicating and conveying information through writing is enhanced by not making it over-complicated. This leads to confusion not clarity. Clarity is also assisted by having a clear structure in what is written and staying focused on the purpose and audience for the writing. Good writing builds credibility and confidence from others. In essence, it is core to and essential within the role of social worker.

Chapter Summary

This chapter considers how competence in writing is central to the role of social workers. It notes how writing skills are embedded and explicit within the HCPC's Standards of Proficiency for Social Workers in England (HCPC, 2012a) and the College of Social Work's PCF (TCSW, 2012). The HCPC also provides a document which shows how the SoP and the PCF are linked (HCPC, 2012b). There is discussion in the chapter of the reasons why writing skills are important and also about the range and relevance of writing requirements for social workers. But overall the chapter's focus is practical – how to write well and how to write specifically for different purposes.

Writing well is of particular relevance if social workers are to perform well in their roles of informing and influencing others and also in being reflective themselves.

Further Reading

- BASW (2012) *How to Deal with Social Media: A BASW (2012) How to Deal with Social Media: A Social Work Union Guide*, available at www.basw.co.uk/resource/?id=782.

- Healy, K. and Mulholland, J. (2009) *Writing Skills for Social Workers*. London: Sage.

- O'Rourke, L. (2010) *Recording in Social Work: Not Just an Administrative Task*. Bristol: Policy Press.

- Seymour, C. and Seymour, R. (2011) *Courtroom and Report Writing Skills for Social Workers*. Exeter: Learning Matters.

References

BASW (2012) *How to Deal with Social Media: A Social Work Union Guide*, available at www.basw.co.uk/resource/?id=782.

Doughty, S. (2014) At Last Victory on Secret Courts, *The Daily Mail*, 17 January: 1.

HCPC (2012a) Standards of Proficiency for Social Workers in England, Health and Care Professions Council, available at http://www.hpc-uk.org/assets/documents/10003B08Standardsofproficiency-SocialworkersinEngland.pdf.

HCPC (2012b) Mapping of the HPC's Standards of Proficiency for Social Workers in England Against the Professional Capabilities Framework – June 2012, available at http://www.hpcuk.org/assets/documents/10003B0BMappingoftheHPC'sstandardsofproficiencyforsocialworkersinEnglandagainstthePCF.pdf.

Healy, K. and Mulholland, J. (2009) *Writing Skills for Social Workers*. London: Sage.

Hill, A. and Shaw, I. (2011) *Social Work and ICT*. London: Sage.

Hopkins, G. (1998a) The Write Stuff: *A Guide to Effective Writing in Social Care and Related Services*. Lyme Regis: Russell House Publishing.

Hopkins, G. (1998b) *Plain English for Social Services: A Guide to Better Communication.* Lyme Regis: Russell House Publishing.

Jones, R., Bhanbhro, S., Grant, R., and Hood. R. (2013) The Definition and Deployment of Differential Core Professional Competencies and Characteristics in Multi-professional Health and Social Care Teams, *Health & Social Care In the Community,* 21 (1): 47–58. ISSN (print) 0966–0410.

Lishman, J. (2009) *Communication in Social Work.* Basingstoke: Palgrave Macmillan.

Ofsted (2010) *Annual Report 2009–10.* London: The Stationery Office.

O'Rourke, L. (2010) *Recording in Social Work: Not Just an Administrative Task.* Bristol: Policy Press.

Peters, T. and Waterman, R. (1982) *In Search of Excellence: Lessons from America's Best-run Companies.* New York: Harper and Row.

Seymour, C. and Seymour, R. (2011) *Courtroom and Report Writing Skills for Social Worker.* Exeter: Learning Matters.

TCSW (2012) Professional Capabilities Framework Domains, *The College of Social Work,* June, available at http://www.tcsw.org.uk/uploadedFiles/TheCollege/CollegeLibrary/ opportunities/professional_practice_development_advisor/domains-within-PCF-May2012.doc.

Truss, L. (2003) *Eats Shoots and Leaves: The Zero Tolerance Approach to Punctuation.* London: Profile Books.

3

PREPARING THE ETHICAL TOOLKIT: BALANCING RIGHTS AND RESPONSIBILITIES

Farrukh Akhtar

Introduction

Every professional has a duty to ensure that their toolkit is appropriately resourced and ready to go. A plumber would be of limited value without a pipe wrench or a doctor without his or her stethoscope. Remember the last time you walked away from an encounter with a professional thinking, 'lovely person, shame they haven't a clue what they're doing'? If we could choose to start off with a clean, empty bag, how would we build a social worker's toolkit?

It would be relatively straightforward to fill it with knowledge of legislation, organisational policies, a range of social work theories, knowledge of local networks and resources. But what about an *ethical* toolkit?

Perhaps more so than other helping professions, good social work depends on the effective 'use of self'. We all have different parts to ourselves. How we behave at work will be different to how we behave with friends or a partner. We may change over time, but there will be a central core, which will remain, defining the essential you. Ward (2010) refers to the self as the primary tool in social work. As with other tools, it requires a worker to learn how to use it effectively. One example is a social worker being able to build a positive working relationship with service users and other professionals, even when those people do not want or see the need for that involvement.

This 'use of self' needs to be carried out in a particular way. Our practitioner may hold up copies of the professional codes and standards that they have signed up to. These may provide important guidelines for their conduct, but they will be of limited use when they are confronted with a difficult situation that needs their immediate attention. In that crucial moment, the choices that a practitioner has are the choice of words: what is said and how, which aspect of the situation is emphasised and the degree with which they can speak with integrity, about their professional position. These are all issues of ethics.

This chapter explores the essential elements needed to build an *ethical toolkit*. It also provides opportunities to review and re-equip an existing ethical toolkit. It is based on the premise that the more self-awareness you have, the more authentically you can carry out your responsibilities. Some of the concepts to be looked at may not be as concrete as a procedures manual, but may prove to be as invaluable.

Practitioners in the early stages of their career often seek clarification around what is ethical and/or professional behaviour. They ponder to what extent their core self needs to embrace their professional self. This can manifest in questions like:

- Is it OK for me to behave in one way at work and another in my personal life? (For example, be responsible for safeguarding the vulnerable at work, whilst being abusive, or being the victim of abuse at home.)

- Can I separate out my religious or political 'self' from my professional 'self'?

- How much of my 'self' do I share with service users? This question is partly around practitioners trying to establish which parts of themselves it is appropriate to reveal in the professional encounter, but it moves beyond a discussion of boundaries. Even the simplest of conversations reveals our value base to others. For example, think about a recent chat you had with someone about a TV programme. How did your comments reflect your value base?

- How do I balance out what a service user needs with my employer's needs and my own need for employment? What do I do if my manager asks me to change the recommendations in my report about a service user because there are no resources available to meet a need, even though the law says it should be met?

- Am I prepared to blow the whistle on dangerous practice, to protect service users, at the risk of losing my job, and perhaps never being able to work as a social worker again?

As this is a skills-based book, rather than detail different ethical challenges, this is done through working with the J family. They will be introduced shortly. Students wanting a more detailed introduction to values and ethics in social work are guided to Akhtar (2013), Banks (2012) and Parrot (2010). Some students find working with case studies frustrating as they can be two dimensional, presenting them with limited information. However, practitioners are expected to work with high levels of uncertainty. They often have to respond to a crisis, being presented with one set of information, only to later find a whole set of other issues as the situation unfolds. The J family's situation will also similarly unfold in the course of this chapter to enable you to think about different aspects of your ethical toolkit.

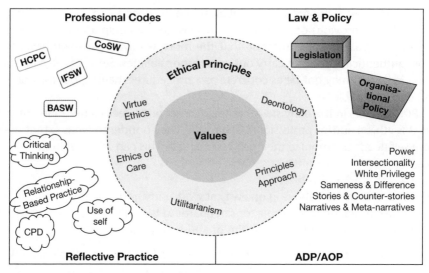

Figure 3.1 The amended values matrix
Source: Amended from Akhtar (2013).

Another way of referring to the different components of the ethical toolkit is to locate them within the framework of a 'values matrix' (Akhtar, 2013) which has been amended and is shown in Figure 3.1.

The matrix shows different dimensions of an ethical toolkit. The examples shown in each domain are just that – examples and not an exhaustive list. The matrix is interactive, with each domain impacting and influencing the others.

The centre of the grid shows how personal and professional values act as lenses through which every other aspect of the framework is interpreted. Ethical theory or principles can act as a buffer between one's values and the other domains, providing a language through which practitioners can articulate and balance out their professional duties and responsibilities from their personal value base. This issue will be explored in more detail later in this chapter. Ethical theories and principles will be discussed and related to the J family.

Professional codes of practice, law and policy form a vital part of the matrix. Whilst the former is signposted, the latter is beyond the scope of this chapter. The two remaining domains (reflective practice and anti-discriminatory/anti-oppressive practice) are also essential to an ethical toolkit. Lack of space precludes a detailed discussion of reflective practice. Fook's framework around critical thinking (Fook and Askeland, 2007) and the model of relationship-based practice (Ruch et al., 2010) are invaluable for those wishing to explore this further. The exercises in this chapter aim to increase awareness of the sense of self so that practitioners can move forward autonomously towards greater reflection in their practice.

Some practitioners use the term 'anti-discriminatory practice' interchangeably with 'anti-oppressive practice' in referring to social-based discrimination (such as on the grounds of race, class, disability, sexuality, age or gender). Others, such as Dalrymple and Burke (2003), define the former as being aware of discrimination and the latter as a means of proactively working to minimise it. The tools listed in this domain are discussed and related to the J family.

This chapter recognises the importance of all of the domains in any ethical toolkit. It focuses on domains relating to values, ethical theory and principles, and to anti-discriminatory/anti-oppressive practice.

Section A explores the development of morality and values which forms the basis of ethical behaviour. Different ethical theories are discussed and related to social work practice. Having established a basic foundation and the central domains of the toolkit, Section B offers tools to enhance anti-discriminatory practice. It begins by looking at concepts of 'sameness and difference' (Akhtar, 2013), the strengths and dangers of each, the nature of individual stories is explored and how understanding a specific experience can provide a clue about wider narratives that a service user may hold about themselves or their situation. There is a closer look at the use and misuse of power in the professional relationship, and the contribution of concepts of intersectionality and white privilege.

Section A: Values, Morality and Ethical Theory

Values and Morality

In beginning to form the foundations of the ethical toolkit, it feels appropriate to start with a consideration of its essential ingredients: values, morals and how they have contributed to the creation of ethical thinking in the Western world generally, and more specifically, within social work practice.

If a value is defined as a standard or behaviour or a fundamental belief about what constitutes right action, then morality can be defined as a system of those values. A worker could believe in the importance of being honest (their personal value) and may exercise this by ensuring that they practice in a transparent way with service users (their sense of morality or professional ethics).

Where do values originate from? How do we develop a sense of what is moral ('right' conduct), immoral ('bad' conduct) or simply amoral (not value-based)? Banks (2008) refers to the elusiveness of values. Thompson (2010) links morality to how an individual makes sense of their wider world. If this is done primarily through a religious framework, then one's morality could be called theonomous (from God). If someone does not have a religious framework and prefers to base their values on their own reasoning alone, their morality has autonomous origins. Those who have elements of both could be said to have heteronomous morality.

For most people, their value base evolves organically without them consciously defining it. Turning implicit values into explicit ones is an essential step in clarifying aspects of our core or essential self.

Reflective Exercise 3.1

What are your most cherished values?

Where do you locate your sense of morality? Is it through theonomous, autonomous or heteronomous means?

Howe (2013) links morality to one's sense of empathy:

Moral codes develop as we balance our own rights and responsibilities against the rights and responsibilities of others. And it is the presence of empathy that ensures that the moral scales are not unfairly tilted.

(Howe 2013: 148)

Howe's (2013) quote is helpful for a number of reasons. For him, having an awareness of one's self is vital to clarifying and perhaps honouring one's own sense of morality and its limits. This is seen as the first step in being able to acknowledge this in others. He emphasises the nurturing of personal attributes, such as empathy in maximising our ability to do this.

Second, the words 'rights and responsibilities' take us from the personal sphere to the professional. They are a reminder that whilst we may all have equal rights our responsibilities will vary with the roles we occupy. Treating a service user with respect may be his or her right, but a social worker may have responsibilities that need to be carried out alongside this, such as an assessment that questions their mental capacity. This may challenge that person's experience of being treated with respect. It is the practitioner's sensitivity and attunement to these issues that will determine the extent to which any 'moral scales' are tilted.

Having a well-equipped ethical toolkit is one way of ensuring that a professional is able to practise in a way that balances individual rights with professional responsibilities. This area is further explored in Section B under the subheading 'Power'.

Introducing the J family

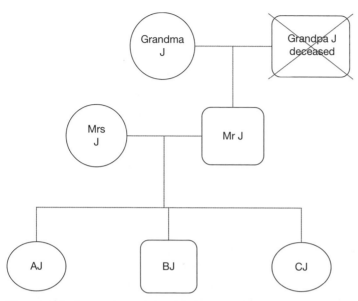

Figure 3.2 Genogram of the J family

Case Study 3.1: **J family: 1**

Mrs J met Mr J when she was 17 years old. He was 35. They got married and moved into the family home. Grandma J had welcomed this as she had lost her husband a few years earlier and did not want to lose her only son as well.

It quickly became apparent to Mrs J that this was a fractious marriage. Mr J would come home drunk and was violent towards her. She had three miscarriages in quick succession. Grandma J was always in her room, apparently unable to hear her if she needed help. Mrs J learnt when to keep out of her husband's way.

Questions

How does this experience of family life compare with yours?

Based on the limited information given, what values do you think are held by the following people about family life?

- Grandma J
- Mr J
- Mrs J

What are your beliefs about family life?

It may be helpful to consider your values; what *should or shouldn't* happen in families? You may have beliefs about the roles and responsibilities of different family members, such as expectations around who does what and where. These may be loose ('it doesn't matter as long as everyone agrees') or rigid ('parents need to … and children need to …').

Why Study Ethical Theories?

The place of theory can often be implicit within social work practice. Ask a practitioner what theoretical approach they use; they are most likely to say they have an 'eclectic' one. Often this means that they are aware of a number of approaches and tend to use different ones in different situations. But it can also imply that a practitioner does not have a sufficient grasp of any theory and does not have a theoretical approach at all. Such practitioners tend to focus on working within a legal framework, ensuring they work within their employer's requirements. They follow the procedures. Theory may seem an academic concept to them.

It is tempting to adopt mechanistic ways of working. Following set guidelines ensures that the work is carried out to organisational requirements, often within tight timescales. The system does not set aside time to think within workload allocations.

Working in this way can be referred to as defensive practice. The worker is defending themselves against the emotional impact of the work. They can no longer cope with managing their caseloads and the feelings this invokes in them. So they lose connection with those feelings.

This may be an acceptable, even necessary attitude to adopt in some professions. A plumber would have a very small business if they let their personal feelings about clients influence their work load too much. But for a social worker to do this would be leaving them open to practising dangerously. As has already been discussed above, social work relies on practitioners having a strong sense of self; this means having an awareness of one's personal 'self' and when this may be helping or hindering the work of their professional 'self'.

This is where having knowledge of an ethical framework can be indispensable. It provides a language through which issues can be articulated and handy short cuts to facilitate decision making.

Ethical Theories and Principles

In thinking about beliefs and values, it is useful to have some knowledge of ethical theories and principles. These were originally devised in an attempt to understand and explain moral behaviour. This section considers a range of different theories (Kantian, Aristotelian, utilitarian, the ethics of care and the principles approach) and applies them to the J family.

Kantian or Deontological Approaches

Immanuel Kant (1724–1804) founded deontology, meaning the duty ('deon') of science ('logos'). Kant was interested in putting forward principles for living that were based on pure logic or reasoning alone. He wanted to distil universal truths that could apply to anyone, anywhere. These he called *categorical imperatives*. These included the following:

- Behaving in a way that you would want others to behave towards you.

- Treating others in a way that respects them, in their own right, rather than in a way that suits you.

In essence, Kant was saying: respect others, don't use them. Treat them as you want to be treated. This focus on respecting others could be said to form the cornerstone of social work, with Kant being referred to as its father.

However, it could be argued that Kant was offering a theory that was quite rigid. One of his categorical imperatives was that we shouldn't lie. If everyone lied, then the whole fabric of society would collapse as it would be impossible for anyone to take another's word at face value. There would be no basis to trust anyone. So, Kant concluded, it was vital to speak the truth, at all times, whatever the consequences. This was a moral obligation.

Reflective Exercise 3.2

What are your views on Kant's categorical imperatives?

Do you always speak the truth, or are there times when you smudge it a little, or lie outright? What are your personal rules about this?

Aristotle and Virtue Ethics

Aristotle (384–322 BCE) lived over 1,700 years before Kant. He had also been concerned about moral behaviour, but his focus was around *eudaimonia* – optimising happiness or enhancing the human soul. Everyone had a responsibility to be the best they could be, by actively working on themselves, developing desirable attributes, minimising undesirable ones. Every citizen needed to contribute to society, depending on these virtues.

Virtue ethics retains relevance in modern life, with its emphasis on personal development, and in social work, with its emphasis on professional capabilities, and continued professional development.

Reflective Exercise 3.3

Which traits or attributes do you most value in yourself or others?

Consider your experience of 'professionals' (your GP or health visitor, dentist, teacher or social worker). What traits do you most value in them?

Read through the Professional Capability Framework (TCSW, 2012) for your level. How do these compare with your views of what attributes are needed for professional practice?

Case Study 3.2: **J family: 2**

AJ was born, followed by the other children. Mrs J focused on raising them. There were periods of relative calm, always followed by an inevitable eruption of violence.

Mrs J did her best to protect her children from their father's temper, but they heard and witnessed much. The results of the violence were frequently seen and heard, but never discussed.

Reflective Exercise 3.4

1 What would deontologoical and virtue ethics have to say about the J family? (Consider Grandma, Mr and Mrs J separately, as well as the needs of the children.)

2 In your view, which theory, if any, offers the most useful framework to consider the J family? Why?

3 What are the limitations of each theory?

Utilitarianism

This theory was founded by Jeremy Bentham (1748–1832) and then further developed by John Stuart Mill (1806–1873). Whilst Aristotle and Kant believed there were correct forms of behaviour, this approach argues that the morality of an action can be judged by its impact on wider society. If an action contributes to the happiness of the majority, it has met its *utility* or usefulness (utility principle).

Utilitarianism promotes liberalism. Anyone can do whatever they like, as long as they don't harm themselves or anyone else (harm principle). Indeed, Bentham and Mill were great emancipators for their time. They argued that homosexuality should be legalised, that women should have the right to vote and that slavery should be abolished.

However, what is seen as the strength of utilitarianism can also be its weakness. Is the reaction of the masses always the best way to determine the 'rightness' of an action? How can the rights of the marginalised ever be recognised if the majority view holds sway?

Reflective Exercise 3.5

1 Name a society in which the minority have been marginalised or oppressed legitimately by the majority.

2 In your view, is this oppression justified?

The Ethics of Care

Gilligan (1993) first put forward her thoughts from a feminist perspective, in the 1980s, arguing that traditional theories do not take into account human beings as social and relational beings, connected and interdependent on each other. They have a need to both give and receive care.

Others have since built on this simple premise to argue from an ethics of care perspective from the micro (i.e. personal) to the macro (i.e. societal) level (Sevenhuijsen, 2000; Tronto, 1993). What has continued to set this approach apart from others has been the emphasis on relationships: everyone has an equal moral worth, and these personal relationships can provide as fertile a ground for moral deliberations as any other. Caring itself is seen as a moral position: how we (as an individual or as a society) care for others and are cared for in return. Caring is seen to enable the growth of the carer, as well as the well-being of those cared for.

Speaking at a macro-level, Sevenhuijsen argues that those in power 'are more often in a position to receive or demand care than to provide it', while those in less powerful positions will be more likely to be providing the care 'without much power over the conditions and the means, and often in positions of invisibility and voicelessness' (Sevenhuijsen, 1998: 24).

At a micro-level, Tronto warns against the powerfulness of the carer in thinking they know more about the needs of those they care for and the inequality that this can lead to.

Care-givers may well come to see themselves as more capable of assessing the needs of care-receivers than are the care-receivers themselves ... especially when the caregivers' sense of importance, duty, career, etc., are tied to their caring role, we can well imagine the development of relationships of profound inequality.

(Tronto, 1993: 170)

Ethics of care has gained much ground; from being seen as a marginal theory, it has become one that connects issues of caring within a global context. However, its critics argue that it still fails to offer guidance about what to do in specific situations.

Reflective Exercise 3.6

What are the different ways that you give and receive care?

Consider those you care for. If power could be quantified as a cake, who holds the largest slice?

Case Study 3.3: **J family: 3**

CJ

When her older siblings (AJ & BJ) were aged seven and two respectively, CJ was born with severe physical and learning disabilities. This meant that she needed and would continue to need a lot of personal care throughout her life.

The diagnosis came at a bad time for Mrs J, who was already suffering from postnatal depression. Grandma J tried to help. However, she had a pre-existing muscular–skeletal condition which became exacerbated. It meant that she had limited mobility and had to start using a wheelchair. Mr J began to stay out for several days at a time.

Reflective Exercise 3.7

1 What would utilitarianism and the ethics of care have to say about Mrs J and her position as a carer within this family? (Consider the strengths and limitations of each theory.)

2 In your view, if power was distributed in a hierarchy in this family, who would have the most, and who would have the least?

The Principles Approach

Another modern ethical 'theory' is Beauchamp and Childress' (2009) 'principles approach' which was first outlined in their seminal text 'The Principles of

Biomedical Ethics' over 30 years ago. As the title of their book suggests, it was written for health professionals, presenting four principles that were said to form the foundation for moral reasoning, each principle being equal to the others. They are as follows:

Autonomy:	To make one's own decision
Beneficence:	To do 'good'
Non-maleficence:	To do no harm
Justice:	Fair and equitable treatment

Within a social work context, it could be argued that students enter the profession because they want to do good and to help others (beneficence). They quickly learn that the helping task is not as straightforward as it was first thought. It involves enabling service users to make their own choices (autonomy) in a way that does not make them dependent on others, protects their rights and the rights of the vulnerable (non-maleficence) and, where possible, balances out social and economic inequality (justice).

The four principles can offer useful parameters when thinking through moral dilemmas, but like the ethics of care, it could be argued that this approach fails to signify the best course of action in any particular situation.

Reflective Exercise 3.8

1 How do the four principles relate to the HCPC Standards of proficiency or The College of Social Work PCFs?

2 In your view, are the four principles equal, or do some principles have a priority over others? (For example, some people would argue that it is more important to prevent harm, than it is to simply 'do good'.) What do you think?

Case Study 3.4: **J family: 4**

Late one night, neighbours called the police after screams were heard from the J family's home.

Mr J had left by the time they arrived, but they found Mrs J bruised and distressed, AJ and BJ hiding in their Grandma's room where she was lying in soiled bedding.

The police noted that the home was in a mess, that there was little food in the kitchen and that Mrs J seemed to be struggling in caring for her baby.

So far we have looked at ethical theories using a case study approach. You may be wondering how relevant ethical theories are to social work practice. You may or may not find them interesting in their own right, but will they really become an essential part of your ethical toolkit?

Progress Check

The College of Social Work PCF in relation to values and ethics states that social workers should 'apply social work ethical principles and values to guide professional practice'.

1   Make a list of the difficulties being experienced by this family.

2   What are the practical steps that could be taken towards resolving these difficulties? Do some actions have more of a priority than others? How do you decide this?

3   How do the four principles apply to any work that might be done with this family? Do any of the principles have a greater priority than any others?

If we go back to your list of difficulties being experienced by the J family, it may look something like this:

- Impact of domestic abuse on each family member.

- Grandma J is bedbound and not able to get to the bathroom.

- Mrs J:

  - is struggling to care for CJ with her complex needs;

  - is suffering from postnatal depression;

  - is not clear to what extent she can protect herself and her children from her husband's violence.

- It is not clear to what extent AJ, BJ and especially CJ are developing within 'normal' milestones and to what extent they may be 'children in need'.

- It is not clear to what extent Mr J acknowledges his behaviour and its impact, and if he is motivated to change it.

In practice, how a practitioner prioritises this list will depend on the agency in which they work and the boundaries of that role. For example, a social worker working in a team for older people would focus on Grandma J's needs whilst a practitioner from a statutory team within Children's Services would prioritise the safety and well-being of the children. A worker from a project dealing with victims of domestic abuse would focus on Mrs J, whilst one from a team working with perpetrators of violence would focus on Mr J.

Whatever specific role a practitioner has, as a minimum, they would need to retain an overall awareness of the family as a whole and the role of other professionals. They would need to consider if anyone is at risk of harm (principle of non-maleficence, utilitarian harm principle), and how they can work in a transparent way that respects every family member (deontology, virtue ethics, ethics of care), their professional remit (principles approach) and their own personal values.

So having an awareness of ethical theories and principles enables shortcuts in thinking, such as being able to ask, *what course of action will enable the greatest service user autonomy, whilst ensuring that no one is at risk of harm?*

Having introduced ethical principles and seen how they can guide professional practice, we now move on to look at aspects of the ethical toolkit that enables practitioners to identify characteristics that promote or hinder effective working with service users: the area of anti-discriminatory practice. This is chiefly referred to in the third PCF (TCSW, 2012); 'diversity: recognise diversity and apply anti-discriminatory and anti-oppressive approaches in practice'. However, there are also some links between this and the following PCF where the mandate is to 'advance human rights, promote social justice and economic well-being'.

Section B: Developing Anti-Discriminatory Approaches in an Unequal World

As a practitioner meeting a service user for the first time, what factors influence your perception of them? One factor will be who you are and the lens through which you see them, and another will be who they are and the lens through which they perceive and so respond to you. In the same way that a camera can focus on different objects bringing some into focus, whilst blurring others, so our assessment of a situation is influenced by the way in which we 'see' it. The tools in this section provide alternative perspectives so that you can diversify the lenses through which you see and therefore work with service users.

Becoming Aware of Sameness and Difference

In Case Study 3.2 you were asked to consider your response to being introduced to the J family and to reflect on your beliefs about family life. Your response to this will vary according to your experience of family life as a child and how you have subsequently made sense of it. You may have witnessed or experienced domestic abuse or it may be so removed from your experience that you might have difficulty connecting to the reality of it. So, the extent to which you feel a degree of 'sameness' or 'difference' (Akhtar, 2013) towards this issue will affect your approach to making sense of it.

There are strengths and weaknesses to each. Yan (2008) found that social workers coming from the same cultural background as their service user found it easier to build a rapport with them. The shared common background was generally seen as a strength, although some service users were afraid that confidentiality was more likely to be breached as a result. Feeling too familiar with a service user, or an aspect of their situation, can also lead to assumptions being made, perhaps even a sense of complacency or over-familiarity.

Working with difference can be just as complex. A positive point is that having no apparent commonality may mean a practitioner has to work consciously to build a constructive working relationship with the service user. However, if they are not careful, they may find themselves struggling to make sense of a situation outside their own experience or comfort zone, and so resorting to broad stereotypes. For example, the belief that domestic violence is more prevalent and therefore more acceptable in some cultures than others or that men from particular cultures are more susceptible to violence.

Reflective Exercise 3.9

In our case study, the J family's cultural background, class and ethnicity have not been specified.

1 In your experience, are some cultures more prone to domestic violence than others?

2 How could this view influence your work with a family suffering from domestic abuse?

If you have answered 'yes', it is helpful for you to be clear about what cultures, in your view, are relevant here; what are the issues of sameness and difference and how would you check them out?

If you have answered 'no', you may feel that you do not discriminate on the grounds of culture or ethnicity and that you treat all service users equally. It may be helpful for you to reflect on how this may impact on the service user: what will it mean for them if you are not able to acknowledge the uniqueness of their situation or their lived experience of their culture?

A concept that can be helpful when considering sameness and difference is the story of the world (Gast and Patmore, 2012) which has its origins in cognitive behavioural therapy. An individual's experiences are interpreted into stories which become internalised into beliefs. For example, a child witnessing one member of the family being repeatedly beaten up by another may internalise the story that the abuse is somehow deserved and that the victim of the violence is worth less than other members of the family.

Being aware of issues of sameness and difference enables individual stories of the world to be unpicked so that a practitioner can arrive at a more authentic sense of a service user's experience. This approach can be further developed by becoming aware of concepts beyond individual stories: those of counter-stories, narratives and meta-narratives.

Becoming Aware of Stories, Counter-stories, Narratives and Meta-narratives

> The stories we select help us ... to interpret the world. They guide us to pay attention to certain things and ignore other things. They lead us to see certain things as sacred and other things as disgusting. They are the framework that shape our desires and goals.
>
> (Brooks, 2009: 24)

Another concept within the story of the world (Gast and Patmore, 2012) is the idea that stories are held collectively and that we behave as if they were true. This can be particularly powerful in national media such as newspapers and television which repeatedly present images of sections of society that then become stereotypes – such as the unemployed scrounging on decent tax payers hard-earned money.

Whilst the story of the world helps to identify a particular story, it can be useful to use the concepts of story, counter-story, narrative and meta-narrative to develop a deeper understanding of a particular situation. Frank (2010) and White's (2004) work are of note here, although I have amended the definitions of generally used terms to the following.

Story

This is the conglomeration of the personal and professional knowledge, beliefs and values that a worker brings to a specific social work encounter, including how they make sense of the service user's situation or the events that led to this encounter.

A social worker visiting the J family for the first time would be bringing a story – their interpretation of the situation which will be based on their preconceptions about the family's background and situation. This may include beliefs about how ineffectual Mrs J is in protecting herself or her family or perhaps locating her in the role of victim.

Counter-story

This is an alternative or opposing account of the story. The term has its origins in critical race theory (Delgado and Stefanic, 2012) which will be discussed in the next section. Here, it refers to the extent that a practitioner can acknowledge the differing realities of each member of a household (while not losing sight of their mandate).

Each member of the J household would have their counter-story about living together, their position within the household and the violence witnessed, inflicted or endured. Without understanding this, it would be difficult for a practitioner to effect change. Mrs J's counter-story could be that her husband is a good man, he is just sick. It is the alcohol that makes him violent.

Narrative

A single story can and often does stand alone. But more often than not, its residue will contribute to a slipstream of hues that merge together to paint a broader landscape.

A child-care social worker, for example, could take Mrs J's apparent faith in her husband as a sign of denial, of her inability to accept the abusiveness of the situation, and therefore her inability to protect her children from harm.

Meta-narrative

Just as a counter-story is an opportunity to present an alternative story or reality, a meta-narrative (also called counter-narrative) can offer the prospect of understanding a service user's wider view of their situation.

Mrs J might not see herself as ineffectual, but rather as someone who is strong and prepared to countenance physical pain to try to keep her family together, for the sake of her children. She might have a broader meta-narrative about the important role of fathers within family life. Unless a practitioner recognises this set of beliefs and works with them, Mrs J may feel alienated and withdraw from the professional encounter.

Allen (2012) offers a helpful narrative approach for working with women experiencing domestic violence. This includes using 'deconstructive questioning' to enable survivors to move from their personal experiences (or counter-stories) to connect with cultural beliefs about women (or their wider meta-narratives), whilst Flood (2008) discusses strategies to redefine manhood as non-violent. Practitioners wishing to use a narrative approach to work with children may find Lacher et al. (2012) useful.

This section has so far looked at how awareness of sameness and difference, stories, counter-stories, narratives and meta-narratives can contribute to understanding discrimination and inequality in the professional relationship. These concepts operate at a personal level and rely on an individual's self-awareness. We now move towards concepts that also include structural and political aspects.

Becoming Aware of Power, Intersectionality and White Privilege

This section looks at different types of power. It then goes on to explore concepts that enable a broader understanding of diversity and social and economic inequality within Western societies: the concepts of intersectionality and white privilege.

Power

Any discussion about discrimination would be incomplete without an acknowledgement of power, its use and misuse. Power can be held in a personal or professional capacity. It can be used in a positive way (reward power) or as a threat (coercive power). It can be acquired through one's position (legitimate power) or through one's experiences, skills or knowledge (expert power). Some people are given power by others as they may be seen to be particularly respected or trustworthy (referent power).

For practitioners to be able to respond justly and fairly, they need an awareness of their own professional power and power within society. Rowson (2006) makes the helpful distinction between being just, which may be about making a plan to fit a specific service user's needs, and being fair which implies that service users are treated appropriately in comparison to others.

Case Study 3.5: **J family: 5**

It is now several years since our last encounter with the J family. Mr J is no longer a part of the household. Grandma J has had adjustments made around the home to enable her to be more mobile as well as having a wheelchair. Her condition has continued to deteriorate. She now lives in the downstairs living room so she can access the bathroom on that floor.

She receives a few hours' personal care a week and one day tells her personal assistant that she suspects Mrs J of stealing money from her purse. She goes on to confide that she regularly hears her hitting CJ and telling her she wished she was dead.

When Mrs J is questioned by social workers, she refutes these allegations, instead accusing Grandma J of spreading malicious lies about her. The personal assistant only visits twice a week. There are times when Grandma J is left waiting for perhaps an hour while Mrs J tends to CJ's medical needs. Mrs J argues that the strain is no longer manageable for her. Grandma J has recently been diagnosed with the early signs of dementia.

Reflective Exercise 3.10

Consider Grandma J, Mrs J and the social worker.
Identify what types of power each has and how they can be exercised.

Thompson's (2012) PCS analysis is useful in taking the discussion of power to a wider level. The P or personal level of discrimination happens at an individual level. At the C or cultural level, discrimination may arise from shared beliefs or attitudes (that might even be unsaid or assumed) within a specific group, such as one's local community or workplace. The S or structural level refers to discrimination at an organisational level within society or within a specific workplace. A company refusing to offer a mini-com facility on the basis that none of their clients are deaf, and being unable to acknowledge that this may prevent deaf users from accessing that service, is one example of this.

If the social worker visiting the J household took a dislike to one or more members of the household, based on characteristics like their gender, race, religion, sexuality and so on, that would represent personal discrimination.

The worker comes from an office where the J family's case has been held for several years. Mrs J has a reputation as being 'difficult and demanding' of resources. So although the practitioner is new to the team and is visiting the family for the first time, they are bringing with them the cultural influences from their workplace (cultural discrimination).

Mrs J has repeatedly argued that the department makes no allowances for her being a multiple carer, and that if Grandma J lived alone, she would be unable to cope on her existing care package. Senior social work managers have made the point that they are providing services in line with their organisational policies and that the family is not eligible to more resources. It could be argued that those policies are set up to discriminate against those with multiple caring responsibilities (structural discrimination).

Tew (2006) distinguishes between the positive and limiting aspects of power, pointing out that used in the right way, it can lead to empowerment (co-operative power) and also the protection of the vulnerable (protective power). Its misuse can lead to collusion with or oppression of service users (collusive and oppressive power).

Reflective Exercise 3.11

The social worker working with the J family decides not to take Grandma J's allegations seriously and not explore them as fully as possible.
What types of power are being used and what are the likely repercussions?

Not all misuses of power are as easy to discern as those outlined above. Sometimes such misuse can be done inadvertently or can result from good intentions. Beckett and Maynard (2009: 116–117) refer to seven further types of unhelpful power. The first of these is social workers' 'exaggerated claims of influence' when the extent of their powers or jurisdiction is over-inflated in an attempt to win over others' co-operation. An example of this would be the social worker promising the J family a transfer to a larger property with disabled access, without first checking out the reality of this.

Next is 'failure of responsibility'. This occurs when practitioners have not fully carried out the duties entrusted to them. The social worker not fully checking out Grandma J's allegations is a good example of this and could lead to them 'neglecting rights', such as those of Grandma J and CJ to be protected and safe from harm.

An 'abuse of position' could happen if, for example, Grandma J's personal assistant started borrowing money from her, with or without the intention of paying her back.

As stated above, not all misuses of power need to be intentional. An example of this is 'disabling help' where a practitioner may be trying hard to get positive outcomes for a service user but may inadvertently be undermining their confidence and perhaps even creating a dependency. This could lead to a specific kind of disabling help – 'undermining personal responsibility' whereby the service user is given the message that they are not responsible for their difficulties, perhaps because of their chronically deprived socio-economic situation or as a result of the abuse they have suffered. If the social worker discovered that Mrs J has been stealing money from her mother-in-law and that she has also been hitting her youngest daughter, instead of working with these issues with the seriousness warranted, she could undermine Mrs J's personal responsibility by making excuses for her.

It can be seen that power is something that is easy to misuse, but if used positively, it also has the ability to create trusting, co-operative relationships that can facilitate change. Practitioners may learn the importance of being aware of discrimination at cultural and structural levels of their organisations and may feel relatively powerless in being able to bring about change here. However, one level that they can influence is at the personal level – that is being aware of their own preferences and tendencies to discriminate against specific groups. To do this, they need an awareness of their own social location in wider society and their responses to others, with the same or different social location. This leads us to the area of intersectionality and white privilege.

Intersectionality and White Privilege

The terms 'intersectionality' and 'white privilege' come from critical race theory, which originated in the United States in the 1970s. Lawyers and legal scholars concluded that they needed a framework that could explain the impact of racism in American society. They postulated that racism is the ordinary everyday experience of Americans of colour. As a social construct, it serves to keep specific aspects of society in advantageous positions, so those in power have little motivation to eradicate it. Rather, different races can be subjected to different racial stereotypes at different times to suit the wider economic needs of society (Delgado and Stefanic, 2012).

Concepts of intersectionality and white privilege were integrated into the theory. White privilege refers to the resulting socio-economic advantages enjoyed by the powerful (mainly white) majority in Western society. Students entering social work training usually have a strong preference to wanting to challenge socio-economic inequality (Fook et al., 2000). Coming across the idea of white privilege for the first time may seem shocking, even offensive, especially if they have a belief that everyone in society is treated equally.

Although critical race theory and the concept of white privilege use race as a starting point, both go on to look at the different points at which individuals can be oppressed – the idea of intersectionality. This takes account of additional forms of oppression (such as gender, sexuality and disablism). It is argued that mapping these intersections enables a more complex discussion about the impact of oppression.

Gast and Patmore (2012) offer a diversity awareness model, in which someone encountering an experience of discrimination (where they may be experiencing oppression, or be the ones who are doing the discriminating) may go through different stages to come to terms with the experience. These follow some of the processes on Kubler-Ross's (2005) stages of grief: moving from a sense of normality, into shock, perhaps denial, before reacting and processing their experience and moving to a stage of acceptance.

Those interested in exploring these concepts further may wish to read Ryde (2009) who writes powerfully from a white perspective about her struggles to understand racism and white privilege. Akhtar (2013) discusses the place of critical race theory alongside other theories of diversity.

The concept of intersectionality can be useful in helping locate possible areas of oppression. However, debates such as 'who is more oppressed, a disabled white man from a middle class background or a black working class policewoman?' may seem academic and contrite. They also do not acknowledge the real struggle that practitioners can have around their own practice, which focuses on wanting to avoid further oppressing clients who may already be disadvantaged through their vulnerable position in society.

For example, how do you assess who is the better long-term parent: the working-class male who is violent towards his partner, is a repeat offender, but is protective of his children, or the partner that is from an ethnic minority background who desperately wants to retain custody of her children but is continually admitted to psychiatric hospital against her wishes for non-compliance of medication?

Of course, we are all more than the sum of our social location and its intersections. But where a service user is at risk of being oppressed by structural, organisational constraints, or by wider society because of the stigma attached to their vulnerability, it becomes especially important for practitioners to think through the ethical issues present and how they have been addressed in their assessment.

Case Study 3.6: **J family: 6**

Sandrine was a single parent who had fought hard to win custody of her daughter from a violent marriage. She came from the same town as Mrs J – Saint Pierre – which was located on the Caribbean island of Martinique.

When she became the social worker for CJ, she identified strongly with Mrs J as a single parent. Mrs J told Sandrine several times that she could no longer manage caring for CJ, who required virtually 24-hour medical care. Sandrine was unable to hear the extent of Mrs J's struggle and the impact this was having on her care of her other children, as well as her own mental and physical health.

Whilst discussing the case in supervision one day, Sandrine was helped, by her manager, to realise that she was putting her own need to keep CJ at home before CJ's best interests. It was difficult for her to accept that she needed CJ to stay at home, more than Mrs J did.

Reflective Exercise 3.12

What are the areas in which Sandrine and Mrs J's lives intersect and how has this impacted on Sandrine's assessment?

(Consider personal and professional intersections and their relevance.)

Conclusion: Balancing Rights and Responsibilities

This chapter has explored the different domains of the values matrix (Akhtar, 2013), including a range of theories and concepts that could form part of a practitioner's ethical toolkit. Table 3.1 lists some of the tools and some practice-based questions to illustrate their use.

Table 3.1 Ethical tools and the related practice-based questions

Tool	Practice-based questions illustrating their relevance
Values matrix	What are my personal and professional values in this scenario? How do I manage to fulfil my responsibilities whilst respecting my personal beliefs and the rights of the service user?
Deontology	What are my duties? How can I carry them out in a way that is respectful to the service user?
Virtue ethics	What attributes do I need to cultivate to be a good practitioner? What is my assessment of this service user's capacity to…?
Utilitarianism	What are the likely consequences of this course of action? What needs to change for the best outcome?
Ethics of care	What is the impact of the caring relationship on the carer and the caree? What are the micro- and macro-care issues?
Autonomy	To what extent can the service user be enabled to make their own decisions and what are the limits to this?
Beneficence	To what extent can I intervene helpfully?
Non-maleficence	What are my obligations to safeguard and protect?
Justice	How can I behave fairly and equitably in this situation? Are my expectations of this service user just and fair?
Sameness and difference	Am I assuming a shared understanding of … because of this similar characteristic? Am I resorting to stereotypes or making unreasonable allowances because this trait or characteristic is beyond my understanding or experience?
Stories and counter-stories	What is my understanding of this event? What is the service user's perception of it?
Narrative and meta-narrative	What does this story contribute to my wider understanding of this case? What can I learn about this service user's understanding of their world, by their interpretation of this situation/counter-story?
Power	How am I exercising power in this situation – helpfully or unhelpfully? What different aspects of power can I use to achieve a positive outcome?
White privilege	Are assumptions around white privilege impacting on the decision making in this case?
Intersectionality	How is my social location and its intersection with that of the service user's impacting on my assessment?

Towards the beginning of the chapter, the issue of rights and responsibilities was raised. Practitioners have responsibility to ensure that they work ethically, in partnership with service users to affect the best possible outcomes for them. But they also have a responsibility to empower service users to take responsibility for their own lives.

This balancing also extends to professionals themselves. They need to ensure they keep in mind their personal and professional selves, taking responsibility for both will prevent burn out in the longer term but will ensure reflective, anti-discriminatory practice in the present.

Chapter Summary

Effective use of self within social work relies on practitioners have a fully functioning ethical toolkit and knowing how to use it to balance rights and responsibilities: for service users and themselves. A values Matrix (Akhtar, 2013) has been introduced as a framework within which such a toolkit could be equipped. It consists of six domains. Some of the tools within those domains have been considered.

Further Reading

- Akhtar, F. (2013) *Mastering Values and Ethics in Social Work*. London: Jessica Kingsley Publishers.

- Gast, L. and Patmore, A. (2012) *Mastering Diverse Practice*. London: Jessica Kingsley Publishers.

- Parrott, L (2010) *Values and Ethics in Social Work Practice*. Exeter: Learning Matters.

  The following websites are interactive and offer useful information on ethics

- The first is the BBC website which can be accessed at: http://www.bbc.co.uk/ethics/introduction/intro_1.shtml Accessed on 25 January 2014

- The second is the Open University Open Learn website. This can be accessed at: http://www.open.edu/openlearn/history-the-arts/culture/philosophy/ethics Accessed on 25 January 2014

References

Akhtar, F. (2013) *Mastering Social Work Values and Ethics*. London: Jessica Kingsley Publishers.

Allen, M. (2012) *Narrative Therapy for Women Experiencing Domestic Violence*. London: Jessica Kingsley Publishers.

Banks, S. (2008) The Social Work Value Base: Human Rights and Social Justice in Talk and Action. In Barnard, A., Horner, N., and Wild, J (eds.), *The Value Base of Social Work and Social Care: An Active Learning Handbook*. Maidenhead: Open University Press.

Banks, S. (2012) *Ethics and Values in Social Work*, 4th edition. Basingstoke: Palgrave.

Beauchamp, T. L. and Childress, J. F. (2009) *Principles of Biomedical Ethics*. 6th edition. Oxford: Oxford University Press.

Beckett, C. and Maynard, A. (2009) *Values and Ethics in Social Work: An Introduction*. London: Sage.

Brooks, D. (2009) The Rush to Therapy, *New York Times*, 10 November.

Dalrymple, J. and Burke, B. (2003) *Anti-Oppressive Practice. Social Care and the Law*. Maidenhead: Open University Press.

Delgado, R. and Stefanic, J. (2012) *Critical Race Theory: An Introduction*. New York: New York University Press.

Flood, M. (2008) Engaging Men: Strategies and Dilemmas in Violence Prevention Education Among Men. In Barnard, A., Horner, N., and Wild, J (eds.), *The Value Base of Social Work and Social Care: An Active Learning Handbook*. Maidenhead: Open University Press.

Fook, J. and Askland, G. A. (2007) Challenges of Critical Reflection: Nothing Ventured, Nothing Gained, *Social Work Education*, 26 (5): 520–533.

Fook, J., Ryan, M., and Hawkins, L. (2000) *Professional Expertise: Practice, Theory and Education for Working in Uncertainty*. London: Whiting and Birch Ltd.

Frank, A. (2010) *Letting Stories Breathe: A Socio-narratology*. London: The University of Chicago Press.

Gast, L. and Patmore, A. (2012) *Mastering Diverse Practice*. London: Jessica Kingsley Publishers.

Gilligan, C. (1993) *In a Different Voice: Psychological Theory and Women's Development*. Cambridge, MA: Harvard University Press.

Howe, D. (2013) *Empathy: What it is and Why it Matters*. Basingstoke: Palgrave Macmillan.

Kübler-Ross, E. (2005) *On Grief and Grieving: Finding the Meaning of Grief Through the Five Stages of Loss*. New York: Simon & Schuster Ltd.

Lacher, D. B., Nichols, T., Nichols, M., and May, J. (2012) *Connecting with Kids Through Stories Using Narratives to Facilitate Attachment in Adopted Children*. London: Jessica Kingsley Publishers.

Parrot, L. (2010) *Values and Ethics in Social Work Practice*, 2nd edition. Exeter: Learning Matters.

Rowson, R. (2006) *Working Ethics: How to be Fair in a Culturally Complex World*. London: Jessica Kingsley Publishers.

Ruch, G., Turney, D., and Ward, A. (2010) *Relationship-based Social Work: Getting to the Heart of Practice*. London: Jessica Kingsley Publishers.

Ryde, R. (2009) *Being White in the Helping Professions*. London: Jessica Kingsley Publishers.

Sevenhuijsen, S. (1998) *Citizenship and the Ethics of Care: Feminist Considerations on Justice, Morality and Politics*. London: Routledge.

Sevenhuijsen, S. (2000) Caring in the Third Way: The Relationship Between Obligation, Responsibility and Care in Third Way Discourse, *Critical Social Policy*, 62: 5–37.

Tew, J. (2006) Understanding Power and Powerlessness: Towards a Framework for Emancipatory Practice in Social Work, *Journal of Social Work*, 6 (1): 33–51.

The College of Social Work (2012) Domains within the PCF, available at http://www.tcsw. org.uk/pcf.aspx, accessed on 25 January 2014.

Thompson, M. (2010) *Understand Ethics*. London: Hodder Headline.

Thompson, N. (2012) *Anti-discriminatory Practice: Equality, Diversity and Social Justice*. Basingstoke: Palgrave Macmillan.

Tronto, J. (1993) *Moral Boundaries: A Political Argument for an Ethic of Care*. New York: Routledge.

Ward, A. (2010) The Use of Self in Relationship Based Practice. In Ruch, G., Turney, D., and Ward, A. (eds.), *Relationship-based Social Work: Getting to the Heart of Practice*. London: Jessica Kingsley Publishers.

White, M. (2004) Working with People Who are Suffering the Consequences of Multiple Trauma: A Narrative Perspective, *International Journal of Narrative Therapy and Community Work*, 1 (1): 45–76.

Yan, M. C. (2008) Exploring Cultural Tensions in Cross-cultural Social Work Practice, *Social Work*, 53 (4): 317–327.

4

WORKING WITH THE EXPERIENCES OF SERVICE USERS AND CARERS

Christine Skilton

Introduction

This chapter will set out briefly the context of service user and carer involvement in social work in the UK and, in particular, how this relates to social work education and practice. It will draw on the perceptions and experiences of those who have been on the receiving end of services and highlight the skills which they consider to be essential in a competent, professional and respected social worker. The benefits of working alongside service users and carers when developing skills for social work will be explained and illustrated through case examples. In considering models of service user involvement in skills development, the chapter will promote the importance of respecting and working with service users and carers from the very beginning of a career in social work and of recognising the expertise that they bring. It will seek to inspire enthusiasm for learning from service users and carers and the confidence to do so.

History and Context of Service User Involvement

Over the last two decades, there has been a drive towards increasing the involvement of those who use social care and health services in their design, delivery and evaluation. These origins of this movement have been located both in the consumerist perspectives of the early 1990s which saw the launch of the Citizens Charter in 1991 (Gordon et al., 2004) and in notions of empowerment prevalent in the mid-1990s (Barnes et al., 2000), and embodied in the government's reform agenda Modernising Social Services (DOH, 1998). This white paper outlined proposals for improving services for adults and for children, in favour of promoting independence and delivering quality services. More recently we have seen a move towards a model of 'stakeholding' and partnership, which acknowledges and values all those who have an interest in an organisation. Although the ideology of service user and carer involvement has its roots in an ethos of 'entitlement' deriving from the Patient's Charter, there is today much more of an awareness of and an emphasis upon human rights, anti-oppressive practice and the promotion of equality in approaches to service user involvement (Gordon et al., 2004).

Turning to service user involvement more in social workers' learning and development, social work education was reformed following the establishment of the General Social Care Council (GSCC) in 2001 (further to the Care Standards Act 2000). Replacing the Central Council for Education and Training in Social Work (CCETSW), the GSCC was given a broader remit to take a lead, not only in education but also in the strategic development of the social care sector in Britain. Although CCETSW had encouraged social work programmes to work closely with service users and carers (CCETSW, 1998), it was the three-year social work honours degree introduced in 2003 that brought with it a mandate for Higher Education Institutions (HEIs) to involve service users and carers in all aspects of the design and delivery of the programme (DOH, 2002). This requirement, which was pivotal in the achievement of a more integrated partnership between education providers and service users and carers, was initially funded by the GSCC, which also published guidance to assist HEIs in developing service user participation (Turner, 2002; Levin, 2004).

More recently, the ongoing support for service user and carer involvement in social work education came into question when the regulation of social workers in England was transferred to the Health and Care Professions Council (HCPC) in August 2012. However, in the event and in accordance with the findings of a commissioned research study (Chambers and Hickey, 2012), the HCPC consolidated the role of service users and carers by introducing a Standard of Education and Training (SET) requiring their involvement in approved qualifying courses.

The emphasis on service user and carer involvement in skills development for social workers has, therefore, evolved from an aspiration to raise standards in service delivery to a professional requisite to counter the potential for their oppression through participative and empowering practice (Molyneux and Irvine, 2004). Besides this, it has been recognised that those who experience a social work service develop an 'expert' knowledge of effective practice through that process (Levin, 2004) from which social workers and training providers can benefit enormously. This recognition is now clearly reflected in the Standards of Proficiency (HCPC, 2012a), the Professional Capability Framework (TCSW, 2012) and the Standards of Conduct, Performance and Ethics (HCPC, 2012b).

What Do We Know About Skills for Social Work and Service User and Carers?

The ability to communicate openly and honestly and to relate to people in sensitive and empowering ways are complex skills that cannot be learnt through reading alone nor can they be taught entirely by academic or practice-based staff. The opportunity to hear from and to work directly with people who have received a social work service, be it positive or negative, adds a further, powerful dimension for skills development (Cree and Davis, 2007). In the context of qualifying training for social work, the Task Force set up by the Social Work Reform Board has made it a requirement for student social workers to undertake 30 days of 'Developing Skills for Practice' (TCSW, 2012) and to be assessed for their 'readiness for direct practice' prior to going out into their first practice learning placement (TCSW, 2012). This 'Developing Skills for Practice' vehicle provides the opportunity for student workshops which concentrate on particular skills, through, for example, role play, case studies, media and interactive materials. The argument made here is that a partnership approach with service users and carers closely involved both in identifying and in teaching skills can be beneficial both to service users and carers themselves and to learners.

There is a developing case in the published literature for the service user and carer contribution to the learning of social work skills. For example, Sadd in the SCIE report 42 (2011) recognises that they are experts in their field and, in common with Webber and Robinson (2012), points to how far they are able to assist students in gaining sensitivity, empathy and insight whilst, at the same time, facilitating the development of reflective practice. Students involved in Wilson and Kelly's (2010) evaluation of the effectiveness of teaching in preparing students for practice learning identified more 'real life' social work practice and more service user and carer involvement amongst those things which might have enhanced their learning (2439). Cooper and Spencer-Dawe (2006) argue that teaching strategies which involve service users and carers representing 'real' life experiences can narrow the gap between theory and practice. For example, a classroom exploration of assessment, whilst seeming a little dry to some, can come alive and gain resonance when recipients of assessments talk of their experiences. We also know from various studies and evaluations that students generally find the involvement of service users and carers enjoyable and effective (Gordon et al., 2004; Cooper and Spencer-Dawe, 2006; Brown and Young, 2008; Skilton, 2011; Webber and Robinson, 2012). Service users and carers also benefit from their involvement feeling that they may be able to improve communication and make a difference to service provision. Although the experience of sharing a personal experience or talking to groups of students can be anxiety provoking and emotionally difficult, service users have expressed their enjoyment of having a valued role, feeling their contributions were appreciated and gaining an increase in their own skills and confidence (Cole, 1994; Frisby, 2001; Gordon et al., 2004; Levin, 2004; Tyler, 2006; Warren, 2007; Brown and Young, 2008; Skilton, 2011).

Finally, we know from various pieces of research and from consultations undertaken across different groups since the 1970s that there is remarkable consistency in what service users value in social workers (Mayer and Timms, 1970; Harding and Beresford, 1996; DOH, 2002; Levin, 2004; TCSW, 2012). The personal qualities and standards of behaviour they expect, in summary, include being supportive, encouraging and reassuring, respectful, patient, committed to the independence of the individual, punctual, trustworthy, open and honest, empathic and warm. Great importance is placed on communication, the ability to listen and the quality of their relationship with the individual social worker. Providing information to service users and carers about services available, assessment and decision making processes and talking 'to' and not talking 'at' or offering any false promises are all attributes rated highly by service users and carers (User Voice, 2010).

Reflective Exercise 4.1

Remind yourself of a situation in your life when you, or someone close to you, may have needed to seek advice or support from a social worker or someone else in a professional position. If you cannot think of anything in the past, consider a situation or a crisis which could happen to you, or someone close to you, in the future. What information would it be important for the social worker or professional person to ask you and what do you think it would be important to tell them?

How would you feel if, rather than hearing this information, the social worker or professional person gave you advice based on their involvement with someone else who had experienced a similar problem previously or from something they had read in a book during their training?

So we know that the ability to communicate effectively and the capacity to develop and maintain positive and compassionate working relationships with people on the receiving end of a 'social work service', whether they are fully receptive or not, is a basic and fundamental skill that social workers must learn. We also have evidence that service users and carers can play a crucial role as we learn these skills. But how can their contribution best be incorporated into the lives of busy students, trainers and social workers?

Models of Service Users' and Carers' Involvement

The concept of service user contribution to the teaching and assessment of social workers, or other care professionals, is not necessarily new, and some higher education institutions involved service user groups in delivering lectures or seminars on an ad hoc basis, prior to the development of the Social Work Degree in 2003. The involvement of patients and service users has been a requirement for pre-registration nursing programmes since 2001 (Nursing and Midwifery Council (UKCC), 2001). Evaluations of the involvement of service users and carers in student learning across professional disciplines have generally been positive, highlighting the value and benefits of learning from those with 'expert knowledge' (Barnes, et al., 2000; Edwards, 2003; Gordon, et al., 2004; Scheyatt and Diehl, 2004; Cooper and Spencer-Dawe, 2006; Collier and Stickley, 2010).

Several authors have supported 'stakeholding' or 'partnership' as the preferred, or more realistic, model underpinning service user and carer involvement as this enables service users and carers to participate as partners whilst, at the same time, acknowledging differentials in power (Taylor, 1998; Barnes et al., 2000; Molyneux and Irvine, 2004). In understanding models and concepts of service user and carer involvement, Arnstein's (1969) 'A ladder of participation', which sets out a continuum of involvement from manipulation to citizen control, has been particularly influential upon those interested in issues of citizen participation. This model was developed in the USA and advocated for the poor or 'have-not citizens' to become more involved in the political and economic processes placing an emphasis on the redistribution of power. However, Arnstein's ladder has been challenged by Tritter and McCallum (2006) as being unhelpfully hierarchical and failing to acknowledge the complexity of user involvement. In a similar vein, it has been argued that an undue focus on power can undermine and detract from the importance and value of service user and carer involvement, which can take place at different levels and have different purposes depending on the context of the involvement (Morrow et al., 2012).

Another continuum of involvement, found useful by authors evaluating service user and carer involvement in student learning (Forrest et al., 2000; Molyneux and Irvine, 2004), works towards the goal of equal partnership, but acknowledges involvement at other levels, and perhaps best recognises some of the complexities in achieving 'full partnership' with equal distribution of power (see Figure 4.1).

Although there is some value in being able to evaluate and measure the level of partnership being achieved, Webber and Robinson (2012: 1257) point out that these continuum models may imply that there is a linear progression towards meaningful involvement whilst actually service user and carer involvement can be meaningful at many levels. Whatever the extent of the involvement, it is recognised that even a small amount of service user and carer input can have 'a dramatic effect on students, making them re-evaluate their preconceptions' (Waterson and Morris, 2005: 659 cited by Brown and Young, 2008).

Level 1: Closed Model – No involvement
The curriculum is defined and delivered with no consultation or involvement of service users

↓

Level 2: Passive Involvement
Based on professional definitions of the issues or problems. Ad hoc service users' views gathered, e.g. through feedback from students or staff

↓

**Level 3: Limited Two-way Communication
(Organisation centred)**
Consultation with service users through non-decision-making forums. Occasional sessional teaching input to organisationally defined curriculum

↓

Level 4: Listening and Responsive
Educationalists listen to user accounts of issues and problems and these form the basis for decisions. Users involved in testing the success of subsequent actions, i.e. curriculum planning and student assessment

↓

Level 5: Partnership
Educationalists and service users work together to identify issues and problems. Open access and involvement of service users at all stages of the planning process. Decisions made jointly. Review and changes undertaken jointly, e.g. assessing students in practice areas, and involvement in research and development projects. Users working as lecturers

Figure 4.1 A continuum of involvement
Source: Goss and Miller (1995).

Providing a Framework

The drawing up of a protocol or working agreement between service users and carers, teaching or training staff and learners which provides a framework around involvement including values, culture, roles and responsibilities, principles, aims and payment policy is valuable in ensuring that all parties involved have the same understanding and expectation (Taylor, 1998; Levin, 2004; Tew et al., 2004). All involved should 'own' the protocol and it must be shared with new learners as they commence the programme. This not only reinforces the importance of service user and carer involvement at the beginning of a programme but also provides information to students about what is expected of them in relation to working with service users and carers during their studies and clarifies expectations around confidentiality and respectful and mature behaviour.

The issue of power also needs to be acknowledged, as the power imbalance between service users and carers and professional staff can raise issues in developing a partnership approach (Hastings, 2000; Edwards, 2003; Molyneux and

Irvine, 2004). Whilst there may be a commitment to seeking, listening to and valuing the views and perspectives of service users and carers, the sharing of power may nevertheless be problematic as it is likely that the academic staff will retain the overall control and power to make final decisions (Barnes et al., 2000). The difficulties in achieving a balance between tokenism and meaningful participation can be partly overcome by generating a planned and structured approach to service user and carer involvement, firmly embedded within the culture of the organisation (Beresford, 1994; Forrest et al., 2000; Turner, 2002; Edwards, 2003). As part of the protocol, educators and trainers need to ensure accessibility for service users and carers, not only in relation to the physical environment but also with regard to the use of language. Their own skills in collaboration and partnership working will be very much called upon. It is quite likely that there will also be service users and carers amongst the staff and student group, and these experiences should be acknowledged and embraced.

Bringing Theory and Practice Together

Social work is about working with people and in developing skills for practice you will be revisiting, and possibly challenging, your our personal values and beliefs. At a personal level, you will be reflecting upon your life experiences and will be considering both how they may assist or inhibit your receptiveness to learning and their potential to impact on your practice. In doing so, you will need to make the link between theoretical frameworks and your concrete experience. At a more general level, you will also be making connections between the organisational and legislative underpinnings of social work practice and direct work with service users and carers. Wilson and Kelly's (2000) study of the effectiveness of social work education highlighted a significant level of disjunction between academic and practice learning and suggested that better integration between these two domains of learning is needed if social work students are to be more effectively prepared for the challenges they are likely to encounter in practice. Service user and carer involvement in your learning can assist you greatly in making these connections as real-life accounts vividly trace the impact of legislation or practice methods on people's lives.

Some programmes involve service user and carer representatives in direct teaching in lectures and seminars, through pre-recorded teaching material or written case studies. Service users or carers may give an account of their own personal situation or background, leading up to and through their involvement with social workers and social care services. For example, their focus might be on experiences of the care system or of mental health services. Service users and carers may share their expertise on direct payments or developments in fostering.

Capitalising on the immediacy of their accounts, service users and carers may also facilitate subsequent student discussion, work with students during learning exercises or be involved in simulated role play exercises.

Service user and carer involvement can be particularly beneficial and influential in learning practice skills. A particularly powerful instance of this is through simulated role play interviews. For example, simulated interviews might form part of an assessment in relation to readiness for direct practice in which all students have the opportunity to interview a service user or carer. Immediate feedback from the service user or carer involved can be supplemented by reflection and self-evaluation on the part of the learner. Where it is possible to record the interview and to play it back, further learning opportunities are created. Published evaluations of this type of exercise highlight the benefits and enhanced potential for learning (Wilson and Kelly, 2000; Moss et al. 2007; Skilton, 2011).

Reflective Exercise 4.2

Imagine you have the opportunity to interview a service user or carer and that you will be observed by a lecturer or a practice educator to assist with your skill development. Consider what skills you think you will need in order to introduce yourself confidently and professionally to the service user or carer, explore the problem they have come to see you about, check with them to ensure you have understood the situation correctly and end the interview competently?

If you then imagine having the opportunity to seek feedback from the service user or carer about how they experienced your approach and intervention, what would you want to know? What questions might you ask? Do you think the feedback may be different from the comments made by the lecturer or practice educator? If so, how and why? How do you feel about seeking feedback and the potential of learning from a service user or carer? How might this change the dynamics in the service user/carer and social worker relationship?

It should not be forgotten that there are opportunities to learn from direct contact with service user or carers in the course of practice itself. During practice placement, students are encouraged and required to seek feedback about their practice, both formally and informally, from a range of the service users and carers with whom they have worked. Those in practice will have other arrangements. Whichever process you have to follow, make the most of the formal and informal opportunities for feedback and evaluation of your practice. In this way, you will create a model of continuous professional development which incorporates the perspectives of service users and carers and gain rich material for supervision and reflection.

Progress Check

If the argument that service users and carers bring an expertise through experience which social workers must draw upon as they develop their skills is accepted, then it will be immediately apparent that their contribution is relevant to a very wide range of skills. Indeed, standard 9.8 of the Standards of Proficiency for Social Workers in England and Wales (HCPC, 2012a) requires social workers to be able to recognise the contribution that service users' and carers' own resources and strengths can bring to social work (P11).

In the same spirit, the Professional Capability Framework (TCSW, 2012), explaining the domain of ethics and values, expects social workers to:

Demonstrate respectful partnership work with service users and carers, eliciting and respecting their needs and views, and promoting their participating in decision-making wherever possible.

Additionally, in respect to knowledge, the PCF requires the development of the ability to:

Value and take account of the expertise of service users, carers and professionals.

This chapter has sought to support readers as they evaluate their current skills in these areas and seek to develop them further.

Ethical Issues

A number of ethical issues are raised by the incorporation of service users and carers into learning programmes. Not least amongst these is their potential vulnerability in a teaching role perhaps unfamiliar to them and potentially disclosing information about themselves and their experiences. To reduce the potential for harm, it is widely recognised (Barnes et al., 2000; Hastings, 2000; Manthorpe, 2000; Levin, 2004; Brown and Young, 2008; Collier and Stickley, 2010) that service users and carers must be offered training and support before and throughout any involvement in a learning and teaching activity and particularly before they share any personal testimonies. The intention must be that service users and carers may be recognised for their expertise and feel empowered through their involvement in the training of social workers and not that the experience is traumatic or exploitative in any way. It is crucial that the organiser or coordinator of any activity is clear with both the service user or carer and the audience about the specific purpose of the involvement, the aims of the session, the context and what will be covered (Manthorpe, 2000; Speed et al., 2012; Webber and Robinson, 2012).

Despite preparation, a service user or carer can become upset on the day, and even if they have shared an experience many times before, they may find themselves overcome with emotion on one particular occasion. Sensitivity and support would be expected from the audience if such a situation occurred and that the organiser takes responsibility for managing the situation. In our experience of this, and in supporting service users after such an event, we find that the service user or carer concerned has been taken by surprise themselves by their feelings, or their sensitivity had been reawakened by another event. It is also the reality when involving and working with service users and carers that crisis occurs and people become unwell, unstable or confused from time to time, so flexibility on the part of the education provider is essential. It again requires sensitivity and understanding if expected service users or carers do not turn up on a particular day when expected or have to leave during a teaching event or exercise.

It is also important to be aware that hearing the personal experiences or testimonies of service users or carers is powerful and can be disturbing. This can resonate with learners' own experiences or evoke feelings around past events lived or witnessed. It is important to prepare for this as far as possible and arrange for appropriate support for the learners. Some may be anxious or feel vulnerable about service users being involved (particularly in their assessment) as there is a shift in the power balance with the service user or carer in this context being overtly in the role of 'expert' (Manthorpe, 2000; Skilton, 2011; Stacey et al., 2011). There may be challenges for both parties in assessed interview situations, with the service user or carers feeling uncomfortable in giving critical feedback and the student defensive in evaluating their own practice and identifying areas for development. These can fruitfully be raised and explored in advance. It has also been highlighted in evaluations and studies that feedback students receive may not be always detailed or consistent, and may be overly positive and not address areas for development. However, general views from students and academics have been positive with students frequently finding service user involvement and feedback rewarding and beneficial (Cole, 1994; Moss et al., 2007; Skilton, 2011; Stacey et al., 2012), enabling them to gain insight into the strengths of their practice and areas for development. Although the organisation of service user and carer involvement is time consuming, and it is not without its challenges, the benefits are well documented and the value added to the programme makes this worthwhile (Barnes et al., 2000; Cooper and Spencer-Dawe, 2006).

Service users and carers appreciate and welcome open and honest feedback from students and lecturers following their involvement in sessions and activities (Crepaz-Keay et al., 1997; Manthorpe, 2000; Speed et al., 2012). This assists with those involved being able to evaluate what has been helpful for student learning and what they may improve upon. At Kingston University, the Service User and Carer Steering Group have devised a pro forma for feedback, and other HEIs or organisations may also have a model.

Case Study 4.1: **Jess**

Jess is 21 years old and has just moved to live independently having been looked after by the local authority since she was 12 years old. Jess was accommodated (Section 20, Children Act 1989) after she found her mother unconscious having taken a drug overdose and she telephoned the emergency services for help. This followed a series of incidents where it had come to light that Jess's mother had taken drugs and alcohol and was unable to care for her children, with her mental health state becoming progressively more fragile. Jess and her younger brother Jason had frequently been left to fend for themselves, with various agencies expressing concern about their health, welfare and lack of school attendance. Jess has come to the university to talk to a group of student social workers about her experiences of social workers and the care system. Jess explains that she has worked with five different social workers since her reception into care and had lived in three different foster placement and two local authority children homes.

You are invited to identify questions you may like to ask Jess about her experiences. Think about the practice skills identified earlier in the chapter and consider what you would hope to gain from this information in assisting your own future practice and professional development. How might you appropriately and sensitively phrase your questions?

Challenges

When evaluating service users and carer involvement, several authors have acknowledged the issue of 'representativeness' in that often service users and carers participating are representing their own views and perspectives based on their own experiences, or of those with whom they have had close contact, and they will of course vary, as the views of professionals vary. However, it is also acknowledged that hearing personal testimonies can have a particular strength in that the experience is conveyed at a personal level and the legitimacy of the view comes from lived experience. It is also not unreasonable to adopt a working assumption that important aspects of one person's social experience will be reflected in the experience of others (Molyneux and Irvine, 2004). It is important to reflect upon the experiences shared and to contextualise them in learning for your own practice, acknowledging that you will be working with a range of views and experiences held both by service users and carers and other professionals.

Some questions arise regarding the diversity of service users and carers involved in learning initiatives. For example, there may not always be the opportunity to hear or consult directly with children in a learning environment, due to the obvious complexities and vulnerabilities involved and the importance of avoiding any further distress or anxiety. However, helpful media resources are available. On the other hand, young people who have experience of the care system are often involved in social workers' training at qualifying and post-qualifying levels.

When involving people with disabilities and communication difficulties, attention should be given to the adaptations which remove obstacles from their path. There are then some excellent learning opportunities for students (Skilton, 2011). The reality is, when developing skills for practice, students will not have the opportunity to hear from or work with every service user and carer group, and the representation from service users and carers from minority ethnic groups has also been recognised as a gap (Sainsbury Centre, 2002).

However, as Beresford (2000) argues, regardless of difference, the key quality that differentiates service user and carer knowledge from all others is that their testimonies alone are drawn from their direct personal experiences of policy, service provision and from being on the receiving end of a social work service (493).

Reflective Exercise 4.3

1 What do you understand by the terms 'service user' and 'carer'?

2 Why do you feel it is important for people who have been on the receiving end of a service to be involved in the teaching and assessment of student social workers?

3 How might this complement the academic curriculum?

4 What ethical actors might you need to consider when working with service users and carers during your social work training?

5 What skills and attributes do you think service users and carers would expect and want from a capable and professional social worker?

Conclusion

The increased emphasis on service user and carer involvement in the education of social care and health professionals recognises that any profession that provides care services needs to be based on a working partnership with people using those services (Hastings, 2000). Although the challenges in achieving a full partnership with service users and carers, rather than 'tokenistic' or 'tick boxing' gestures (Tyler, 2006), are significant, it was acknowledged by Forrest et al. (2000) over a decade ago that we had come a long way, and it is apparent from the range of published literature that we have come further still since then. If the ultimate aim of involving service users and carers is to improve the way in which services are provided so that they are more effective in meeting the needs of those in receipt of them (Levin, 2004; Molyneux and Irvine, 2004; Tyler, 2006), then it is crucial to involve service users and carers at an early stage in social work education (Levin, 2004). Developing effective skills for practice needs to take place alongside the gaining of insight into service user's and carer's personally felt experience. Teaching and learning activities where the knowledge and expertise of service users and carers is incorporated alongside theoretical input enhance student learning (Scheyett and Diehl, 2004; Cooper and Spencer-Dawe, 2006) and assist in developing communication, support interpersonal skills and challenge power imbalances. Although there are challenges when involving service users and carers in social work education, ultimately there is strong evidence to support the fact that it enriches the curriculum, with the ultimate aim to improve social work practice and the outcomes for service users and carers themselves (Webber and Robinson, 2012).

Chapter Summary

This chapter has argued that service users and carers have a vital role to play in the development of social workers' practice skills. It has traced the history of the contribution made by service users and carers to social workers' learning and has identified models of collaboration between learners, educators and service users and carers. Ethical issues and organisational challenges have been addressed and the development of the skills which might benefit most from engagement with service users and carers has been identified.

Further Reading

- Crepaz-Keay, D., Binns, C., and Wilson, E. (1997) *Dancing with Angels*. London: Central Council for Education and Training in Social Work.

  This practical handbook makes some points which are of relevance to seeking the views of service users generally and acknowledges that although the involvement of, in this case, mental health survivors, does entail additional time, their contribution offers 'a unique and crucial perspective to training' (p. 2).

- Skilton, C. J. (2011) Involving Experts by Experience in Assessing Students' Readiness to Practice: The Value of Experiential Learning in Student Reflection and Preparation for Practice, *Social Work Education*, 30 (3): 299–311.

  This paper reviews the development of an experiential learning exercise, designed to involve service users and carers in assessing students' readiness to practice. This article draws out some of the strengths and advantages of involving 'experts by experience' in helping students to develop an awareness of self and of effective communication skills, ultimately promoting the importance of reflective practice early in their training. It also acknowledges some of the problems and dilemmas in providing an equitable experience to students when involving service users and carers.

References

Arnstein, S. (1969) A Ladder of Citizen Participation, *Journal of the American Institute of Planners*, 35 (4): 216–224.

Barnes, D., Carpenter, J., and Bailey, D. (2000) Partnerships and Service Users in Interprofessional Education for Community Mental Health: A Case Study, *Journal of Interprofessional Care*, 14 (2): 189–199.

Beresford, P. (2000) Service Users' Knowledges and Social Work Theory: Conflict or Collaboration?, *British Journal of Social Work*, 30: 489–503.

Beresford, P. with Page, L., and Stevens, A. (1994) Changing the Culture: Involving Service Users in Social Work Education, CCETSW Paper 32.2, London: Central Council for Education and Training in Social Work.

Brown, K. and Young, N. (2008) Building Capacity for Service User and Carer Involvement in Social Work Education, *Social Work Education*, 27 (1): 84–96.

Central Council for Training & Education in Social Work (1998) Conference on Promoting the Involvement of Service Users in Education and Training for Social Work and Social Care, New York, 11 November.

Chambers, M. and Hickey, G. (2012) Service User Involvement in the Design and Delivery of Education and Training Programmes Leading to Registration with the Health Professions Council, available at www.hcpc.org.uk

Cole, A. (1994) 'It was an education' Service Users Assess Student Social Workers, *Community Living*, (16–17 January).

Collier, R. and Stickley, T. (2010) From Service User Involvement to Collaboration in Mental Health Nurse Education: Developing a Practical Philosophy for Change, *The Journal of Mental Health Training, Education and Practice*, 5 (4): 4–11.

Cooper, H. and Spencer-Dawe, E. (2006) Involving Service Users in Interprofessional Education Narrowing the Gap between Theory and Practice. *Journal of Interprofessional Care*, 20 (6): 603–617.

Cree, V. E. and Davis, A. (2007) *Social Work: Voices from the Inside*. London: Routledge.

Crepaz-Keay, D., Binns, C., and Wilson, E. (1997) *Dancing with Angels*. London: Central Council for Education and Training in Social Work.

Department of Health (DOH) (1998) *Modernising Social Services*. London: The Stationery Office.

Department of Health (DOH) (2002) *Requirements for Social Work Training*. London: Crown.

Edwards, C. (2003) The Involvement of Service Users in the Assessment of Diploma in Social Work Students on Practice Placements. *Social Work Education*, 22 (4): 341–349.

Forrest, S., Risk, I., Masters, H. and Brown, N. (2000), Mental Health Service User Involvement in Nurse Education. *Journal of Psychiatric and Mental Health Nursing*, 7: 51–57.

Frisby, R. (2001) User Involvement in Mental Health Branch Education: Client Review Presentations. *Nurse Education Today,* 21, 663–669.

Gordon, F., Wilson, F., Hunt, T., Marshall, M., and Walsh, C. (2004) Involving Patients and Service Users in Student Learning: Developing Practice and Principles, *Journal of Integrated Care,* 12 (6): 28–35.

Goss, S. and Miller, C. (1995) *Margin to Mainstream: Developing User and Carer Centred Community Care.* York: Joseph Rowntree Foundation.

Harding, T. and Beresford, P. (1996) *The Standards We Expect: What Service Users and Carers Want from Social Services Workers.* London: National Institute of Social Work.

Hastings, M. (2000) User Involvement in Education and Training. In Pierce, Rachel and Weinstein and Jenny (eds) *Innovative Education and Training for Care Professionals.* London: Jessica Kingsley.

Health and Care Professions Council (2012a) *Standards of Proficiency.* London: HCPC.

Health and Care Professions Council (2012b) *Guidance on Conduct and Ethics for Students.* London: HCPC.

Health & Care Professions Council (2013) Consultation on Service User Involvement in Education and Training Programmes Approved by the Health and Care Professions Council (HCPC), available at http://www.hcpc-uk.org/assets/documents/10004110 Consultationsonserviceuserinvolvementineducationand trainingprogrammes-consult ationresponsesanddecisions.pdf.

Levin, E. (2004) *Involving Service Users and Carers in Social Work Education.* Bristol: SCIE, Policy Press.

Manthorpe, J. (2000) Developing Carers' Contributions to Social Work Training, *Social Work Education,* 19 (1): 19–27.

Mayer, J. E. and Timms, N. (1970) *The Client Speaks: Working Class Impression of Casework.* London: Routledge and Kegan Paul.

Molyneux, J. and Irvine, J. (2004) Service User and Carer Involvement in Social Work Training: A Long and Winding Road?, *Social Work Education,* 23 (3): 293–308.

Morrow, E., Boaz, A., Brearley, S., and Ross, F. (2012) *Handbook of Service User Involvement in Nursing and Healthcare Research.* West Sussex: Wiley-Blackwell.

Moss, B. R., Dunkerley, M., Price, B., Sullivan, W., Reynolds, M., and Yates, B. (2007) Skills Laboratories and the New Social Work Degree: One Small Step Towards Best Practice? Service Users' and Carers' Perspectives, *Journal of Social Work Education,* 26 (7): 708–722.

Sadd, J. (2011) *'We are more than our story' Service User and Carer Participation in Social Work Education,* SCIE report 42 Online, available at www.scie.org.uk.

Sainsbury's Centre for Mental Health (2002) *Breaking the Circles of Fear: A Review of the Relationships Between Mental Health Services and African and Caribbean Communities.* London: The Sainsbury Centre for Mental Health.

Scheyett, A. and Diehl, M. J. (2004) Walking Our Talk in Social Work Education: Partnering with Consumers of Mental Health Services, *Journal of Social Work Education,* 23 (4) 435–450.

Skilton, C. J. (2011) Involving Experts by Experience in Assessing Students' Readiness to Practice: The Value of Experiential Learning in Student Reflection and Preparation for Practice, *Social Work Education,* 30 (3): 299–311.

Speed, S., Griffiths, J., Horne, M. and Keeley, P. (2012) Pitfalls, Perils and Payments: Service User, Carers and Teaching Staff Perceptions of the Barriers to Involvement in Nursing Education. *Nursing Education Today,* 32, 829–834.

Stacey, G., Stickley, T., and Rush, B. (2012) Service User Involvement in the Assessment of Student Nurses: A Note of Caution, *Nurse Education Today,* 32: 482–484.

Taylor, I. (1998) *Developing Learning in Professional Education. Partnerships for Practice.* Buckingham: Open University Press.

Tew, J., Gell, C. and Foster, S. (2004) Learning from Experience Involving Service Users and Carers in Mental Health Education and Training: A Good Practice Guide, Higher Education Academy, National Institute for Mental Health in Higher Education. Trent Workforce Development Confederation, Nottingham.

The College of Social Work (2012) *The Professional Capabilities Framework.* London: TCSW. Online, available at tcsw.org.uk/pcf.aspx.

Tritter, J. and McCallum, T. (2006) The Snakes and Ladders of User Involvement: Moving Beyond Arnstein, *Health Policy,* 76 (2): 156–168.

Turner, M. and Shaping Our Lives National User Network (2002) Involving Service Users in Social Work Education: Southampton, Social Policy and Social Work Learning and Teaching Support Network (swapltsn), available at www.swap.ac.uk.

Tyler, G. (2006) Addressing Barriers to Participation: Service User Involvement in Social Work Training, *Social Work Education,* 25 (4): 385–392.

United Kingdom Central Council for Nursing, Midwifery and Health Visiting (2001) *Requirements for Pre-registration Nursing Programmes.* London: UKCC.

User Voice (2010) Does Social Work Care?: A User Voice consultation for the College of Social Work, The College of Social Work and Centre for Innovation in Health Management, University of Leeds, available at www.uservoice.org.

Warren, J. (2007) *Service User and Carer Participation in Social Work.* Exeter: Learning Matters.

Webber, M. and Robinson, K. (2012) The Meaningful Involvement of Service Users and Carers in Advanced-Level Post_qualifying Social Work Education: A Qualitative Study, *British Journal of Social Work,* 42: 1256–1274.

Wilson, G. and Kelly, B. (2010) Evaluating the Effectiveness of Social Work Education: Preparing Students for Practice Learning, *British Journal of Social Work,* 40: 2431–2449.

5

ASSESSMENT FOR SOCIAL WORK PRACTICE

Rick Hood

Introduction

Arguably, almost everything social workers do is connected to assessment in some way. Indeed, it is such a fundamental part of social work that any discussion of assessment could easily turn into a recital of the entire social work skill-set. Clearly this is beyond the scope of this chapter, which will focus instead on what makes assessment a discrete and distinctive activity. The first section will examine what is generally meant by assessment and will introduce the main principles that underpin social work practice in this area. The second half of the chapter will then explore what social workers need to know and do when carrying out assessments in a variety of settings, including preparation and planning, gathering information and using research to inform conclusions and recommendations. Some case examples are presented from relevant service areas, such as adult social care, child protection and mental health.

What is Assessment?

Assessment has been variously defined in the social work literature. For example, Walker and Beckett (2011) consider it to be about helping people 'to identify areas for growth and change' (2) and also note that it involves establishing a 'problem-solving partnership' with people. Taylor and Devine (1993) refer to assessment as part of a 'basic helping cycle' (2), along with planning, implementation and review. Others have developed the idea of assessment as a precursor to intervention or as part of a process in which interventions are planned, carried out and then evaluated (e.g. Sutton, 1999; Thompson, 2005). In the UK, this view of assessment as a distinct activity has arguably been promoted by reforms to the welfare state over recent decades. In the field of adult social services, for example, social workers help to control access to care provision by carrying out an assessment of eligibility based on government guidelines. On the other hand, it has also been pointed out that assessment can be 'a service in its own right' (Whittington, 2007: 29), such as when courts request a report from the local authority as part of private family proceedings.

A frequently cited model is that of Milner and O'Byrne (2009), who developed a five-stage approach to assessment:

- preparing for the task;

- collecting data;

- applying professional knowledge;

- making judgements;

- deciding and/or recommending what is to be done (2009: 4).

This model has the advantage of providing a practical-sounding template that fits in with the workflow common to many social work settings. However, Milner and O'Byrne caution against assuming that assessment is a straightforward process of gathering data and reaching objective conclusions. Social workers are likely to come across several versions of 'the truth' during the course of an assessment, each offering pragmatic benefits and drawbacks to different people. Assessment takes place within an interpersonal, institutional and socio-political context, and this includes the power dynamics that emerge when people disagree about what the problem is and what kind of change is desirable. Practitioners therefore need to be vigilant about how they develop, confirm and challenge their own judgements, and accept and manage a degree of uncertainty, however uncomfortable this may feel (White et al., 2006). This is partly a reflection of the complex and unpredictable reality of professional practice, which has memorably been compared to 'a swampy lowland in which situations are confusing "messes" incapable of technical solution' (Schön, 1991: 42). It is also a consequence of trying to work in partnership and build relationships with clients rather than impose the social worker's own view of their problems and strengths.

Principles of Assessment

Assessment can therefore be seen as a set of joint activities that begin the process of change. It may even be the social worker's only contribution to that process. All the elements of change, including strengths and capacities as well as problems and difficulties, are negotiated through dialogue and interaction. In negotiating this complex territory, it is important for social workers to bear some fundamental principles in mind. In what follows, three such principles will be described: working in partnership, reflective practice and ethical decision-making.

Working in Partnership

The term 'partnership' suggests that the working relationship between those involved in an assessment should be based on mutually respectful interactions and a sense of shared involvement and responsibility. This invites us to consider the power dynamics between practitioners and service users, as well as with parents, carers, family members and professionals from other agencies. In this respect, Smale and Tuson's (1993) discussion of three models of assessment may help to dissect some of our assumptions about power, expertise and participation.

The first is what Smale and Tuson (1993) call a 'procedural model', in which eligibility for services is determined using a checklist of criteria supplied by the agency. This model limits the role of service users to that of providing information – they have no say over the decision that is made. Practitioners have a limited form of discretion, which may allow them to 'advocate' for resources by interpreting information in a particular way that leads to criteria being met. The second model of assessment discussed by Smale and Tuson is a 'questioning' model, in which the main task is to collect information that enables the specific situation to be analysed via the practitioner's own knowledge base. The service user's role is to provide 'data' that is relevant or useful to the chosen framework. Milner and O'Byrne (2009) suggest that this model of assessment is often used in conjunction with the 'procedural' type, especially when questions of risk are being addressed.

What Smale and Tuson (1993) call the 'exchange model' of assessment promotes the ability of service users to define their own needs and strengths in order to initiate problem-solving. Here it is the practitioner's approach to relationship-building that leads to positive and sustainable change. The onus is on following up the 'leads' provided by the service user rather than the presumption that the practitioner will know best. This requires a careful and empathetic approach to communication, using open questions and inviting the service user to tell their story. Similar ideas have informed the application of an anti-oppressive perspective to the assessment process (Dalrymple and Burke, 2006).

Power imbalances between professionals, agencies and service users are often exacerbated by broader social inequalities. This means, for example, that children from deprived areas are much more likely to be taken into public care than children from affluent areas (Bywaters, 2015), while people from black and minority ethnic backgrounds are over-represented among service user groups such as in-patients on psychiatric wards (Bowers et al., 2009). Differences in socio-economic status, gender, culture and class identity may also be prominent in practitioner–service user relationships. Practitioners must work hard to bridge gaps in knowledge and understanding, especially in statutory settings where the failure to work appropriately with diversity can lead to abuses of authority. The ability to communicate and understand information across cultures is therefore crucial at all stages of assessment. Equally, there may be particular challenges involved with working from someone from the 'same' culture (see Fontes, 2008).

In summary, some basic principles to remember are as follows:

- Assessments are carried out with people, not 'of' or 'about' them.

- The practitioner's approach should be honest, open and respectful at all times.

- The institutional and statutory context of the assessment should be explained.

- Differences between service users and practitioners should be acknowledged and an effort made to bridge gaps in knowledge.

- Where there are concerns, criticise the problem and not the person.

- The viewpoints of all those involved in an assessment should be represented in the assessment.

- Conclusions should be transparent, including why decisions were made and what alternative options were considered.

- Write any reports in a clear and accessible way.

Reflective Practice

As we shall see in Chapter 8, the term 'reflective practice' covers a key set of skills that social workers employ in all areas of practice. In their assessments, social workers are often being asked to judge complex situations and deal with uncertainty, which requires a high degree of self-awareness and a conscious dialogue between intuition and analysis. Keeping a 'reflective mindset' (O'Leary et al., 2013) allows the practitioner to:

- Apply systematic principles to the process of learning from experience.

- Be explicit about the theoretical models and frameworks they are using.

- Question the influence on their professional judgement of 'common-sense' assumptions and preconceptions.

- Actively make and test hypotheses as part of assessment and intervention.

- Remain open to the positive role of emotion, while recognising the impact of stress and anxiety.

- Recognise and address the power dynamics in their relationship with service users and others.

However daunting the above list might appear, the underlying principles are indispensable. No matter how busy they are, social workers have to make time to think carefully about what they do, how they are doing it and why they are choosing to do it in a particular way. In this respect, Schön (1991) has drawn an oft-cited distinction between 'reflection-on-action', which occurs after an activity has taken place, and 'reflection-in-action', which takes place during the activity itself. He surmises that the latter is characteristic of more experienced professionals. Other commentators have differentiated between 'reflection', 'critical reflection' and 'reflexivity' (see D'Cruz et al., 2007, for an overview), although such distinctions are not developed in this chapter. In particular, the reflective learning cycle associated with writers such as Kolb (1984) is familiar to most social workers (see Chapter 8). Its basic principle is to think about a situation that has occurred, draw out significant aspects of the experience, make the link to generalised concepts and then apply what has been learnt to a new situation. The cycle is continuous and can be embedded in individual supervision as well as practice development in social work teams.

In relation to assessment, reflective practice has particular implications for the way social workers analyse information and come to decisions. As Munro (2008) and others have pointed out, the divide between intuition and analysis is often overplayed, as is the distinction between practice wisdom and 'academic' theory. Both are involved in making judgements about complex situations. Experienced social workers may well be able to grasp swiftly what is going on in a given situation, but still make sure to check their initial assumptions. For example, a social worker may be concerned that the elderly man she is visiting is depressed. To begin with, this judgement will be an intuitive one, based partly on her observations of the man's appearance or way of speaking, along with what he might disclose about his activities, thoughts and feelings but also drawing on her accumulated knowledge about the causes and symptoms of mental illness. At the same time, by helping the service user to complete a validated questionnaire such as the Beck Depression Inventory (Beck et al., 1988), she will acquire further evidence to confirm or contradict her analysis. Relying on intuition alone ignores the limitations of personal experience and the possibility of bias (Munro, 2008).

Ethical Decision Making

Skills for ethical practice were discussed in Chapter 3. Here the focus is on how social workers draw on ethical principles and frameworks in their decision making. It could be argued that the whole purpose of assessment is to make decisions. Even before their formal conclusions and recommendations, assessments present a series of judgements about the significance of information and its implications for people's welfare and safety. Arguments about the nature of problems, and the strengths and resources available to address them, take shape during the assessment process and may to differing degrees take account of disagreements and uncertainties. In social work assessments, such judgements are usually framed as decisions about *need* and *risk*. From a developmental perspective, the concept of need concerns the conditions that are necessary for human growth and well-being, including the fulfilment of personal goals (e.g. Maslow, 1968). From a professional point of view, a shortfall in these necessary conditions suggests a 'need' for assistance and support. Such ideas also tend to be embedded in statutory definitions. For example, Section 17 of the 1989 Children Act defines a 'child in need' in terms of whether optimal health of development will occur without the provision of services. In addition to identifying areas of need, social workers are usually required to assess the degree of need, which means evaluating their impact on a person's health and welfare. The predictive element to needs assessment is related to the concept of risk, which formally involves a calculation of the severity and probability of a given outcome (Munro, 2008). It is worth noting that this does not necessarily mean an adverse outcome, although this is how risk is commonly understood.

Decisions about need and risk may be complicated by ethical dilemmas, as illustrated by the example below.

Case Study 5.1: **Peter**

Peter is an 85-year-old man who has Crohn's disease, a condition that requires him to manage his diet carefully. He also suffers from chronic arthritis, which is making it increasing painful to do basic household chores. He lives alone and has no close family living nearby. He has requested home help to assist him in cooking and cleaning the house. However, the social worker conducting the assessment knows that his current level of need is not enough to make him eligible for this service.

In the case of Peter, the social worker will probably understand and sympathise with Peter's wish to have some level of home help. She may even believe that the local authority's eligibility criteria are too strict, as they do not allow for people like Peter to receive assistance until their condition deteriorates to the extent that their health is seriously impaired. Nonetheless, she is required by her professional and institutional role to make sure that resources are allocated fairly and efficiently, bearing in mind that there is always a scarcity of services relative to need. As Walker and Beckett (2011) point out, such dilemmas are characterised by a clash between *deontological* and *utilitarian* ethical philosophies. Deontological ethics concern the moral duties that people perceive in particular situations, for example to help someone whom we think requires assistance. Utilitarian ethics, on the other hand, requires us to consider the overall consequences of our actions, and this might mean withholding a service from some people if others will benefit more from it. A feature of many social work settings, particularly in the statutory sector, is that decisions about resources are made by managers, so that frontline social workers are often in the position of requesting or advocating for services on behalf of their clients. This may have the advantage of simplifying the ethical burden on practitioners and managers alike, but at the expense of structural inconsistency in how the organisation behaves towards its service users. For example, some practitioners might perceive a duty to secure services for 'their' clients by allocating them to a higher category of need than would be the case if eligibility were not restricted. Likewise, some managers might feel that budgetary constraints outweighed human rights considerations in individual cases.

If decision making sounds like an ethical minefield, it is worth remembering that social workers are not expected to 'get it right' in every assessment. As with other aspects of their work, professional accountability lies in basing one's judgements on sound principles of thought and action that can be evidenced and documented. The decisions you take as a social worker should therefore demonstrate the following:

- Transparency, e.g. being clear about the methods you have used and your reasons for making a decision;

- Integrity, e.g. articulating the service user's perspective, acknowledging areas of disagreement and uncertainty;

- Expertise, e.g. using a variety of assessment tools, using research evidence to justify assertions;

- Consistency, e.g. making sure that you apply similar criteria across individual cases.

Assessment Skills: Knowledge and Method

Having established some of the fundamental principles of assessment, we will now address the specific elements of expertise that constitute a social work assessment. In other words, what is it that social workers need to know and do in order to carry out an effective assessment? In considering this question, we must bear in mind that assessment is a cyclical as well as linear process. Knowledge and method are interdependent, since what we know constantly changes and informs what we do and vice versa. On the other hand, assessments have a definite beginning and end point, which requires the social worker to organise their knowledge and methods in a structured way. This cyclical integration of assessment skills is illustrated in Figure 5.1.

Again it is worth emphasising that assessments will often resist the attempt to follow a strict chronological order. Assessment is a complex process, all the

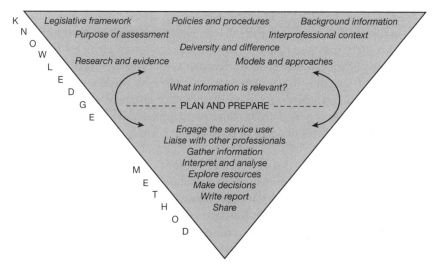

Figure 5.1 The assessment process: knowledge and method

more so when the messy reality of families' lives starts to intrude on what professionals might wish to address or accomplish. Indeed professional involvement itself may influence the situation in unpredictable ways (Reder et al., 2005). As new information comes to light, the purpose and direction of assessments might change entirely. Practitioners also need to be wary of adhering too rigidly to a plan of work, as this may lead them to misinterpret or ignore information that does not fit in with their perceived ideas. Nonetheless, to simplify the discussion, it is proposed to look at each of these elements in turn, using illustrations from some of the different settings in which social workers operate.

What Social Workers Need to Know

LEGISLATIVE FRAMEWORK   What is the legal remit for your assessment? Many social workers are employed within statutory agencies, in which their roles and functions stem directly from primary legislation. For example, a social worker who has completed the training to work as an approved mental health practitioner (AMHP) may be asked to judge whether someone's mental health has deteriorated to the extent they should be admitted to hospital for assessment under the 1983 Mental Health Act. The social worker may well be based in a multi-disciplinary community mental health team (CMHT), and so her responsibilities as an AMHP will constitute only a small part of the legal framework governing the activities of the team. Nor is mental health legislation the only relevant body of law. The same social worker may be responsible for coordinating care for another patient who has been discharged from hospital and faces eviction from their property. This will require a working knowledge of homelessness legislation, such as the provisions set out in the 1996 Housing Act and the Homelessness Act 2002. Awareness of the Equality Act 2010 may also help mental health practitioners advocate for patients and provide guidance on reasonable adjustments for employers (Lockwood et al., 2012). And it is not only in the statutory sector that the legal context to assessment is important. Social workers in voluntary sector organisations play a vital role in providing services to vulnerable children and adults and in making referrals to statutory services in cases of acute need or where there is a risk of abuse.

POLICIES AND PROCEDURES   The format and content of social work assessments is nowadays shaped by procedures set out in national and local guidelines. Social workers carrying out a child protection investigation, for example, will follow the protocols in *Working Together* (Department for Education, 2013) as well as local guidelines (e.g. London Safeguarding Children Board, 2013). Social workers carrying out community care assessments currently apply local thresholds to eligibility criteria on adult care and support, although national criteria may soon be adopted (Department of Health, 2013). Agencies will usually have their own policies and templates for implementing the guidance. In child and family social work, statutory assessments are undertaken on a variety of computerised forms conforming to the Integrated Children's System (ICS), which explore specific areas of need and capacity (Shaw et al., 2009). In mental health settings, social workers will be using a national system, the Care Programme Approach (CPA), in order to assess and manage complex needs. Particularly in the statutory sector, social workers will have timescales and deadlines for when assessments should be completed. It is also important to bear in mind that policies and procedures can change quickly as new legislation and guidance comes into effect. It is therefore essential for social workers to keep up to date on the procedures relevant to their work, for example by subscribing to a professional journal, making use of online resources and attending relevant training.

BACKGROUND INFORMATION   You will doubtless meet social workers who prefer 'not to know anything about the client' before they first meet them, so as not to prejudice their views of the person or the situation. This sounds plausible but is in fact discrediting the practitioner's ability to practice reflectively and hold different perspectives in mind. Adopting a 'tabula rasa' approach to assessment is more often than not a response to time pressure, i.e. not having (or making) time to read the file. The problem with this is that practitioners may be selective about their subsequent file reading, having been influenced by their impressions of the initial meeting or visit. Of course, the amount of background information can vary enormously between assessments. There may only be a few lines in a faxed referral, or social workers may have access to an entire case file including previous assessments, chronologies, medical reports, statements of educational needs and other professional records. Depending on what is available, social workers may be able to gain quite a comprehensive picture of the service user and their life or they may not even have basic demographic information such as age and ethnicity.

Background information is important in planning and preparation and allows the social worker to anticipate potential challenges and identify gaps in their own knowledge and expertise. Chronologies are particularly useful in risk assessments in order to identify patterns and avoid 'start-again syndrome' (Brandon, 2009). Service users who have had previous professional involvement will also appreciate not having to repeat their whole story to another stranger or explain why a particular treatment has failed in the past. Assessing risk also includes the personal safety of professionals and students, particularly (but not exclusively) in relation to service users who have been aggressive or violent in the past. Safety planning might consider issues such as the timing and location of visits, co-working arrangements, 'buddy systems' and supervision requirements.

Purpose of Assessment   What does a social worker do? What is an assessment and what is it for? It is tempting for social workers simply to assume that their service users know these things, not least because they can actually be quite tricky to explain. However, knowing and being able to explain the purpose of assessment is a crucial first step for establishing working relationships. There is a big difference between telling somebody that you are there 'to assess their needs' before producing your 20-page form or asking somebody what they are hoping to get out of your visit. Surprisingly often, the latter question will elicit confusion about what you are doing there in the first place! Social workers also have to find ways of explaining what they do without using jargon or alienating language – for example to young children, people with learning difficulties or those recently arrived from another country. If there are safeguarding concerns, explaining the purpose of the assessment allows social workers to be clear about what they are worried about and highlights the 'signs of safety' that will begin the process of addressing those concerns (Turnell and Edwards, 1997).

Inter-professional Context   Social workers must work in partnership not only with service users but also with other professionals. Social workers usually work in a multi-agency context, and this is particularly the case when aspects of risk and need are being assessed. Social workers will rely on other professionals for crucial aspects of the assessment – for example the diagnosis of physical and mental illness, the nature and extent of disability or the necessary steps to enable rehabilitation and recovery. Carers and support workers will have in-depth knowledge of the service user's needs that the social worker lacks. Resources and services recommended by the assessment will often be carried out by non-social work agencies. Social workers should also be prepared to coordinate multi-agency assessments in safeguarding cases or as part of integrated health and social care teams.

DIVERSITY AND DIFFERENCE   As we saw earlier, the principle of working in partnership means paying close attention to issues of diversity and difference right from the start of the assessment. Holland (2010) suggests undertaking a 'cultural review' before our first contact with a service user (see also Dalzell and Sawyer, 2007). The review involves a structured series of questions that help us to examine our knowledge and assumptions about people from a particular cultural background or life experience. The idea is to explore some of the unconscious influences on the way we understand and engage with families. It includes asking ourselves how a particular family will perceive us – as professionals, as representatives of a particular agency or as members of a particular socio-economic class or majority/minority group. We should consider what impact the assessment might have on the family's life or what might surprise us about this particular family and why (Dalzell and Sawyer, 2007: 21). Having reflected on these questions, we should then consider what action we need to take, e.g. to discuss particular issues in supervision, consult a colleague with 'insider' knowledge of a subject or undertake a joint home visit with another professional.

Undertaking a review of this sort should also help clarify some of the process issues inherent in conducting assessments with people across cultures. This includes the practical aspects of setting up meetings, such as deciding who you need to speak to and in what setting. It is worth reviewing your usual communication style as a professional, considering issues such as body language, how you establish rapport, whether to address people by their first or last names, how many and what type of questions to ask, methods of greeting and leave-taking and so on. Working with interpreters creates a series of separate issues around selection, preparation and conduct of interviews, which need to be considered in advance (Fontes, 2008).

MODELS AND APPROACHES   As noted earlier, there is a strong procedural aspect to social work assessments in most settings. Nonetheless, there remains ample scope for professional discretion in the way they are conducted. Most social workers will have a preferred set of ideas, a conceptual toolkit to help them interpret and address some of the most common problems in their client group. This may mean an allegiance to a particular model of understanding and changing human behaviour in a social context. Social workers tend to be familiar with the following general approaches:

- psychodynamic;
- behavioural or cognitive-behavioural;
- task-centred;
- solution-focused.

Milner and O'Byrne (2009) present a useful overview of these models and their implications for assessment. For example, social workers adopting a cognitive-behavioural approach will focus on identifying not only the problematic behaviour that the service user wishes to change but also the beliefs and self-perceptions associated with that behaviour. In contrast, a solution-focused approach looks ahead rather than at the past; service users are encouraged to draw out the characteristic elements of a 'problem-free' future as a way of identifying and building on the resources necessary to achieve that goal. Depending on the background information available, social workers may prefer to begin the assessment without making a firm decision about which model to use. On the other hand, they or their agency may specify a particular framework – such as the 'Signs of Safety' approach for child protection cases. In any event, social workers need to be able to explain to their services users what approach they are adopting and why.

Many social workers will maintain an eclectic attitude to the general frameworks mentioned above. Nonetheless, even eclecticism will eventually manifest itself in a preferred way of working, as social workers begin to draw on their practice experience as well as more specialised theoretical knowledge. In time, their expertise in certain areas may be acknowledged by their agency, either as a formal role or as an informal agreement to be allocated in certain types of case. Examples of such specialisms might include child sexual exploitation or adults with dual diagnosis of mental illness and substance misuse. As social workers begin to specialise in this way, they will become familiar with other models and approaches, such as systemic family therapy or domestic violence prevention. Such expertise is hugely valuable to social work teams and enables assessments to be tailored to specific problems and needs. Equally, social workers should be wary of assuming that their favoured way of working will always be the most useful or relevant one.

RESEARCH AND EVIDENCE Newly qualified social workers are often surprised to hear senior practitioners say that they 'do not use' research in their assessments. This is unlikely to be true, as experienced professionals have been found to integrate a variety of formal and informal knowledge when judging complex situations and making decisions (White et al., 2006). The statement instead reflects a common perception that 'practice' and 'theory/research' are fundamentally separate worlds, whose only intersection lies in qualifying and post-qualifying courses. Yet an assessment is similar in many respects to a piece of social research, in terms of the ethics of professional conduct as well as the methodological process. The ability to explore and critically evaluate the literature on a particular topic is a very useful skill for assessments. For example, social workers may wish to look at the research evidence for:

- prevalence and common causes of a problem;
- susceptibility within particular groups and communities;

- risk factors that are predictive of illness, maltreatment or social exclusion;
- effectiveness of a treatment or intervention;
- particular models of service provision.

Referring to the evidence base on such issues helps to establish a clear basis for the analysis. Managers may also be more inclined to authorise funding for a resource if the social worker has been able to point out the cost-effectiveness of alternatives. Of course, this does not mean that assessments should read like academic essays; no one is going to thank you for that!

WHAT INFORMATION IS RELEVANT?   This question may be seen as the starting point for investigation, after the social worker has comprehensively reviewed the areas outlined above. Considering relevance does not mean closing off potential areas of inquiry but is about being clear about what you want to find out and why. In some respects, this is as much an ethical issue as a practical concern; after all, social workers should not be conducting a 'fishing expedition' into people's lives, on the off-chance that what they discover might come in useful. Relevant information is often guided by statutory guidance and assessment frameworks or may be linked to the preferred approach of the practitioner. A social worker may decide to carry out an adult attachment interview as part of an assessment of suitability for adoption, for instance. It is also worth considering what evidence might be useful to confirm *and to refute* the social worker's working hypotheses, e.g. about the presenting problems or the nature of risks.

What Social Workers Need to Do

PLAN AND PREPARE   Planning and preparation should ideally encompass all of the areas discussed above. By way of illustration, consider the following scenario:

Case Study 5.2: **Evser**

Evser is a 20-year-old Kurdish woman who came with her parents to the UK six years ago from Turkey. She is five months pregnant. Evser lives in a flat with Recep, the father of her unborn child. At an antenatal appointment, the community midwife notices some bruises on her arms. Evser discloses to the midwife that Recep hits her sometimes when he has been drinking. A referral is made to the hospital social work team, and following a strategy discussion it is decided to carry out a pre-birth assessment including Section 47 inquiries in respect of the unborn child. The case is co-allocated to a social work student and her practice educator.

Even from this brief outline, you should be able to describe several relevant areas of knowledge. In terms of legal framework, the 1989 Children Act confers powers and duties on the local authority to undertake inquiries when there are concerns about future risk of harm to the unborn child. Other areas of legislation that may be relevant in this case include human rights, domestic violence and immigration law. Social workers must adhere to the protocols for completing core assessments and convening multi-agency meetings, e.g. child protection conference to be held ten weeks (at the time of writing) before the expected delivery date. The assessment itself is likely to cover pre-defined categories, including risk factors, strengths in the family environment and potential areas of change (see Calder and Hackett, 2013). The inter-professional context is very important in cases like this, with the social worker likely to work closely with the police, health services and community organisations.

Reflective Exercise 5.1

Using the case example of Evser described above, think further about your planning and preparation. How would you work with issues of diversity and difference? Do you have a model or approach in mind? What research and evidence could help to inform your assessment? What information is particularly relevant here?

ENGAGE THE SERVICE USER   However brief it may be, the relationship between practitioner and service user is one of the most important factors in an effective assessment. It can also be one of the most challenging. Social workers often get only a few 'brief encounters' (Kohli and Dutton, 2010) in which to address a range of complex issues. People's reaction to a visit from a social worker may be evasive, fearful, angry or despairing, and these emotions will inevitably trigger a response in the worker. Practitioners will confess to feeling relieved on the odd occasion when a knock on the door goes unanswered! In undertaking an assessment, social workers are mindful of having 'a job to do' that relies to a large extent on the other person's motivation and contribution. The process of 'engaging' a service user in an assessment is therefore highly skilled work.

Martin (2010) summarises some of the interpersonal skills required by social workers, including non-verbal communication, active and empathetic listening, and the use of open questions. Such skills are particularly important when dealing with people who are reluctant or resistant to participating in the assessment. As noted earlier, social workers need to adapt their own communicative needs to those of service users, including people who speak little English or who might find it difficult to take part in a meeting or interview. Social workers often employ particular methods to communicate and carry out direct work with children and young people (Luckock and Lefevre, 2008). Combining formal assessment methods with participation in simple, everyday activities, such as going to the park or even for a drive in the car (Ferguson, 2011), can be a way of superseding the bureaucratic and professional barriers to building a relationship. Cases of potential abuse or neglect present a particular challenge in this regard. In undertaking their inquiries, social worker will need to carry out investigative interviews that put an emphasis on purposeful interaction. This type of interview demands particular skills, such as the ability to interpret body language and detect patterns of inconsistency and ambiguity in the interviewee's responses (see Martin, 2010: 35).

LIAISE WITH OTHER PROFESSIONALS/AGENCIES   Social work assessments will generally draw on the contribution of a range of professionals, often (though not exclusively) working in sectors such as health, education, social care, housing, criminal justice and the police. Communicating with these professionals is essential to gain an understanding of the service user's situation and the associated needs, strengths, resources and risk factors. Social workers therefore need to build an inter-professional approach into their assessments from the start (Hammick et al., 2009). Who are the other people in the network? What are their contact details? What will they want or expect from you as the social worker? In safeguarding cases, the social worker will have a coordinating role and other professionals will need to be fully involved in the process of analysis and decision making. Social workers will be expected to keep their colleagues updated with developments and make sure that dates and venues for meetings are discussed and shared in advance.

It is also worth thinking about what type or degree of collaboration is preferable in each case. For example, the service user may already have a positive relationship with another professional, such as a health visitor, key worker or mentor. These relationships may prove to be a key resource in the assessment. Joint visits or meetings can be a useful way of making introductions, alleviating service user's wariness or anxiety and obtaining a 'second opinion' about specific issues or observations. Equally, there may be tensions in the relationship between service users and other professionals or between professionals themselves. Social workers will need to be mindful of these dynamics when they are liaising with other agencies. This includes maintaining an open and respectful attitude on their part towards unfamiliar working practices and organisational cultures. Other professionals may not immediately see the need to share confidential information about their client, for example, or even to return a social worker's phone calls. The reverse also applies, and due to their coordinating role in safeguarding matters, social workers often have a particular responsibility to liaise with other professionals.

GATHER INFORMATION Social workers base their assessments on information obtained from a number of sources, including the background information as discussed already. Hepworth et al. (2010) note the following methods of gathering information:

- interviews with service users;

- direct observations (including non-verbal behaviour and interactions between people);

- self-monitoring by the service user (e.g. occurrence of particular events and feelings);

- information obtained from family members, friends and other professionals;

- assessment instruments and questionnaires;

- the practitioner's own experience of interacting with the service user (2010: 181).

Of these different sources, interviews are perhaps the most commonly used. Carried out effectively, interviews should enable the service user to present their own account of their circumstances, while also allowing practitioners to draw out the relevant information. It is skilled work that requires social workers to establish a rapport, demonstrate empathy for the other person's feelings, respect their dignity, probe important points and verify that they understand what is being said. Interviews with some service users, such as children, may require more specialised techniques and resources. However, even the most informative interview will be influenced by unconscious bias and inaccurate recollection, on the part of practitioner and service user alike. Interviews should therefore be supplemented by other sources of information.

Observational learning, including the practice of observation-based analysis and reflection, has become an established part of social work training. Its significance for assessment should not be underestimated. Paying attention to body language and non-verbal cues can provide useful detail to back up the judgement of emotional state or psychological functioning. A record of interactions, for example between a parent and child at a supervised contact session, often forms part of the basis for later decisions and recommendations. Social workers may ask service users to 're-enact' particular situations or events, so they can gain a more complete picture of what happened, or set up 'contrived situations' that encourage service users to model their approach to stressful activities or decision making (Hepworth et al., 2010: 182). Social workers also have the opportunity to visit people at home, which may reveal strengths and needs that are not necessarily reported. Observation is therefore an important aspect of safeguarding work, and social workers may even be diverted or discouraged from accessing certain areas of the home (Ferguson, 2011).

Another way of obtaining information is through 'assessment instruments', which are questionnaires with established reliability in testing for the presence or severity of particular problems. Such assessments are often administered by doctors or psychologists, but others have been developed for use by a range of health and social care professionals. For example, the Department of Health produced a 'Family Pack of Questionnaires and Scales' as a specific resource for social workers assessing children in need and their families (Cox and Bentovim, 2000). These questionnaires can help practitioners evaluate problems such as drug and alcohol misuse or domestic violence. On the other hand, social workers need to be cautious about using 'off-the-shelf' questionnaires without first researching the evidence for their reliability and perhaps consulting with other professionals as to how to administer them.

INTERPRET AND ANALYSE INFORMATION   It should already be evident that a key principle in assessment is 'triangulation', a term used by researchers to refer to the combination of different methods, observers or theoretical approaches to enhance their understanding of a phenomenon. This is an important principle to bear in mind when it comes to analysis. It is important to recognise that interpretation is not a discrete, individual activity but is a social process that is constantly taking place throughout the assessment. Social workers must remain open to new information, and to the views of others, in order to hold alternative hypotheses in mind. At the same time, analysis is bound up with the purpose of assessment and the framework being used to identify problems, risks, needs and strengths. Social workers should therefore be clear about what they are hoping to achieve through their analysis. One way of doing this is illustrated in the exercise below:

Reflective Exercise 5.2

Consider the following types of assessment. What are the key questions that your analysis would need to answer?

- A residential parenting assessment of a couple with a three-year-old daughter and a history of substance misuse.

- A pre-sentencing report on a 15-year-old boy who has sexually assaulted a 20-year-old woman.

- A carer's assessment of an 80-year-old man whose wife has severe mobility problems.

In answering these questions, social workers will probably want to clarify risk and protective factors in relation to a particular problem, such as child abuse or criminal behaviour, but will also consider how the interaction of a given cluster of factors affects the *overall* pattern of likely events. As discussed earlier, there has been something of a false dichotomy in social work between 'intuitive' and 'analytical' thinking, with an emerging consensus that analysis actually requires a synthesis of both. Adopting a systematic approach to analysis makes it easier to explain and justify the decisions that are made. In this respect, Calder and Hackett (2013) outline some general principles of risk analysis in child care assessments, which can also be adapted to other settings:

- What are the 'weaknesses' in the situation, i.e. factors that make the occurrence or continuance of the problem more likely?

- What are the strengths and protective factors in the situation?

- What are the prospects for change in the situation and for growth?

- What can be offered to build on strengths and address weaknesses?

- What are the risks associated with potential interventions?

- What is the service user's motivation and capacity for change?

- What is the overall level of risk or need? (Calder and Hackett, 2013: 13–14)

Milner and O'Byrne (2009) point out that part of the analysis process should involve testing any preliminary explanations for the situation. This means checking with service users and other stakeholders in the assessment, such as the professional network, whether (or which) explanations seem most accurate or plausible. In keeping with the reflective approach advocated here, it is also advisable to review *all* the information obtained in the light of the theoretical framework adopted for the analysis. Have any pieces of information been overlooked, or interpreted a particular way, in order to make them 'fit'? What other explanations could be developed at this stage?

EXPLORE RESOURCES AND INTERVENTIONS   A crucial part of the assessment is developing a plan of action based on the analysis of problems, strengths and needs. Social workers should be clear about their reasons for recommending a particular intervention, its purpose and how a successful outcome is to be gauged. Interventions tend to follow the approach taken for the assessment itself. For example, a social worker may have had discussions with a service user about the possible links between their violent behaviour and negative feelings, such as shame or anger. From a cognitive behavioural standpoint, the intervention might then encourage the service user to recognise and record the negative feelings at the points when they occur and practise alternative ways of responding to them. From a psychodynamic perspective, on the other hand, the intervention might involve counselling or psychotherapy sessions to assist the service user in coming to terms with difficult or abusive experiences earlier in life. A risk management approach would also require some sort of safety plan in order to protect the welfare of vulnerable family members. It is important to establish whether the resources to carry out the intervention are available in an acceptable time-frame. This may involve getting authorisation or funding agreement from managers, or establishing the waiting time between referral and initial appointment, before making your recommendations.

MAKE DECISIONS AND RECOMMENDATIONS Decision making may be regarded as the final stage of analysis, in which a reasoned choice is made between alternative explanations and courses of action. This can be a stressful process for practitioners, who may be worried about 'getting it wrong' and being blamed for adverse outcomes. However, it is worth remembering that professional accountability lies in the competence and integrity of the activity carried out, rather than the outcome on its own, and that all decisions carry an element of risk. What is important is that the rationale for decisions is clear and reasonable, given the available information and state of professional knowledge at the time. In relation to child protection assessments, for example, Munro (2008) advocates a systematic approach and the use of analytical tools such as 'decision trees'. Such tools enable practitioners to evaluate possible decisions by considering both the utility of potential outcomes as well as the probability that such outcomes will occur. Taking the time to work through such exercises enables social workers to clarify their thinking and arrive at an informed decision.

WRITE AND SHARE THE REPORT Even when there is ongoing social work involvement, most assessments result in some form of written report that is shared with service users, carers and other professionals. This is an important document, with potentially far-reaching consequences. Social workers should therefore approach the task of writing with the same respect and consideration they would demonstrate in a face-to-face meeting. Reports should use language that is accessible to those who will be reading it, which means avoiding jargon and explaining technical terms where necessary. It is also important that service users and carers are invited to read the assessment, or have the opportunity to comment on its contents, before it is disseminated to others and placed on file. Taking time to do this enables inaccuracies to be corrected and wording to be adjusted, which can often save aggravation in subsequent meetings.

Progress Check

The skills discussed in this chapter should help you to undertake assessments of need and risk (SoP 1.3), and identify people's rights, strengths and capacities in what are often challenging circumstances (PCF 7.4). Carrying out effective assessments is essential in order to identify and respond to signs of abuse and neglect (SoP 1.5, and PCF 5.7). This means being able to collate relevant information (SoP 14.1), work within procedural multi-agency frameworks (PCF 8) and analyse and critically evaluate what you know, in order to inform your decisions and recommendations (PCF 6.2).

Conclusion

Social work is a diverse field, covering a range of regulatory contexts and practice settings. The process of assessment will vary accordingly and so it has been possible only to provide a broad outline in this chapter. Particularly for social workers at the beginning of their careers, assessment can seem a daunting task and it is usually helpful to work in a structured and systematic way. The skilled practitioner will be able to develop a thoughtful combination of knowledge and methods in each individual case. Of course, there is never an exact methodology or 'blueprint' for carrying out assessments, which is precisely why the social worker's expertise and judgement is required. As always in social work, it is important to stick to fundamental principles, while making sure the assessment matches the unique circumstances of the service user and fulfils the professional's remit and responsibilities. Students and practitioners are therefore encouraged to draw on the guidance and literature in their own area of specialisation.

Chapter Summary

- This chapter explores the importance of assessment skills in social work practice. Assessment can be viewed as a set of joint activities that begin the process of change. Strengths and capacities, as well as problems and difficulties, are negotiated through dialogue and interaction with the service user.

- Social workers carrying out assessments need to work in partnership with others, engage reflectively with the complex situations they encounter and make decisions in an ethical and accountable way.

- Assessments usually have a timescale for completion, as they may contribute to statutory or organisational frameworks of intervention. This means social workers have to plan and organise their work in a structured way, without becoming too rigid in their approach.

- Knowing and doing are inextricably linked in the assessment process, in that social workers must hold uncertainty while they formulate and test hypotheses, look for relevant information and evidence and record their analysis in support of conclusions.

- A vital part of assessment is inviting service users to comment on and contribute to the written report before it is placed on file or shared with others.

Further Reading

- Calder, M. and Hackett, S. (2013) *Assessment in Child Care. Using and Developing Frameworks for Practice*, 2nd edition. Lyme Regis: Russell House Publishing.

  A detailed and comprehensive guide to assessments in child protection, safeguarding and family support.

- Mandelstam, M. (2008) *Community Care Practice and the Law*, 4th edition. London: Jessica Kingsley.

  A comprehensive guide to community care assessments and the legal frameworks, including case law. A 'quick guide' covering similar ground is also available from the same author.

- Milner, J. and O'Byrne, P. (2009) *Assessment in Social Work*. Basingstoke: Palgrave Macmillan.

  An accessible overview of the assessment process, including sections on each of the main social work approaches.

- Parsloe, P. (1999) *Risk Assessment in Social Care and Social Work*. London: Jessica Kingsley.

  This edited volume provides an introduction to the concept of risk and explores risk assessment in fields such as offenders, older people and mental health.

References

Beck, A., Steer, R., and Carbin, M. (1988) Psychometric Properties of the Beck Depression Inventory: Twenty-five Years of Evaluation, *Clinical Psychology Review*, 8 (1): 77–100.

Bowers, L., Jones, J., and Simpson, A. (2009) The Demography of Nurses and Patients on Acute Psychiatric Wards in England, *Journal of Clinical Nursing*, 18 (6): 884–892.

Brandon, M. (2009) Child Fatality or Serious Injury Through Maltreatment: Making Sense of Outcomes, *Children and Youth Services Review*, 31 (10): 1107–1112.

Bywaters, P. (2015) Inequalities in Child Welfare: Towards a New Policy, Research and Action Agenda, *British Journal of Social Work*, 45 (1): 6–23.

Calder, M. and Hackett, S. (2013) *Assessment in Child Care. Using and Developing Frameworks for Practice.* Lyme Regis: Russell House Publishing.

Cox, A. and Bentovim, A. (2000) *Framework for the Assessment of Children in Need and Their Families: The Family Pack of Questionnaires and Scales.* London: TSO.

Dalrymple, J., and Burke, B. (2006). *Anti-oppressive practice: Social care and the law* (2nd Edition). Maidenhead: Open University Press.

Dalzell, R., and Sawyer, E. (2007). *Putting Analysis into Assessment.* London: National Children's Bureau.

D'Cruz, H., Gillingham, P., and Melendez, S. (2007) Reflexivity, its Meanings and Relevance for Social Work: A Critical Review of the Literature, *British Journal of Social Work*, 37 (1): 73–90.

Department for Education (2013) *Working Together to Safeguard Children.* London: TSO.

Department of Health (2013) *Draft National Minimum Eligibility Threshold for Adult Care and Support: A Discussion Paper.* London: TSO.

Ferguson, H. (2011) *Child Protection Practice.* Palgrave Macmillan: Basingstoke.

Fontes, L. (2008) *Interviewing Clients Across Cultures.* New York: Guilford.

Hammick, M., Freeth, D., Copperman, J., and Goodsman, D. (2009) *Being Interprofessional.* Cambridge: Polity Press.

Hepworth, D., Rooney, R.., Rooney, G., Strom-Gottfried, K., and Larsen, J. (2010) *Direct Social Work Practice: Theory and Skills*, International edition. Belmont, CA: Cengage Learning.

Holland, S. (2010). *Child and Family Assessment in Social Work Practice* (2nd Edition). London: Sage.

Kohli, R. and Dutton, J. (2010) Brief Encounters: Working in Complex, Short-term Relationships. In Ruch, G., Turney, D., and Ward, A. (eds), *Relationship-based Social Work: Getting to the Heart of Practice.* London: Jessica Kingsley.

Kolb, D. A. (1984) *Experiential Learning Experience as a Source of Learning and Development.* New Jersey: Prentice Hall.

Lockwood, G., Henderson, C., and Thornicroft, G. (2012) The Equality Act 2010 and Mental Health, *The British Journal of Psychiatry*, 200 (3): 182–183.

London Safeguarding Children Board (2013) *London Child Protection Procedures and Practice Guidelines.* London: LSCB.

Luckock, B. and Lefevre, M. (2008) *Direct Work: Social Work with Children and Young People in Care.* London: British Association for Adoption and Fostering.

Martin, R. (2010) *Social Work Assessment.* Exeter: Learning Matters.

Maslow, A. H. (1968) *Toward a Psychology of Being*, 2nd edition. Princeton, NJ: Van Nostram.

Milner, J. and O'Byrne, P. (2009) *Assessment in Social Work.* Basingstoke: Palgrave Macmillan.

Munro, E. (2008) *Effective Child Protection.* London: Sage.

O'Leary, P., Tsui, M.-S. and Ruch, G. (2013) The Boundaries of the Social Work Relationship Revisited: Towards a Connected, Inclusive and Dynamic Conceptualisation, *British Journal of Social Work*, 43 (1): 135–153.

Reder, P., Duncan, S., and Gray, M. (2005) *Beyond Blame: Child Abuse Tragedies Revisited.* London: Routledge.

Schön, D. A. (1991) *The Reflective Practitioner: How Professionals Think in Action.* Aldershot: Avebury Academic Publishing.

Shaw, I., Bell, M., Sinclair, I., Sloper, P., Mitchell, W., Dyson, P., and Rafferty, J. (2009) An Exemplary Scheme? An Evaluation of the Integrated Children's System, *British Journal of Social Work*, 39 (4): 613–626.

Smale, G., and Tuson, G. (1993) *Empowerment, Assessment, Care Management and the Skilled Worker*. London: National Institute for Social Work.

Sutton, C. (1999) *Helping Families with Troubled Children*. Chichester: Wiley.

Taylor, B. J. and Devine, T. (1993) *Assessing Needs and Planning Care in Social Work*. London: Arena.

Thompson, N. (2005) *Understanding Social Work*. Basingstoke: Palgrave Macmillan.

Turnell, A. and Edwards, S. (1997) Aspiring to Partnership. The Signs of Safety Approach to Child Protection, *Child Abuse Review*, 6 (3): 179–190.

Walker, S. and Beckett, C. (2011) *Social Work Assessment and Intervention*. London: Russell House Publishing.

White, S., Fook, J., and Gardner, F. (2006) *Critical Reflection in Health and Social Care*. Maidenhead: Open University Press.

Whittington, C. (2007) *Assessment in Social Work: A Guide for Learning and Teaching*. London: Social Care Institute for Excellence (SCIE).

6

APPLYING THEORY IN PRACTICE

Wilson Muleya

Introduction

The chapter begins by defining the terms 'social work theory' and 'social work practice'. This leads on to a discussion of the role of theory in social work and how theory is applied in practice where I look at eclectic practice and evaluate the effectiveness of this approach. Drawing on this background, I propose a fishbone framework as an alternative expository approach for applying theory in practice. The proposed framework aims to enable practitioners to maximise the effectiveness of selected theories and incorporate research evidence leading to best practice in their assessments and interventions and to further develop their practice skills. The discussion draws on case examples from a range of service areas to illustrate the key aspects. The chapter ends with a conclusion and makes reference to professional standards.

Social Work Theory

Social work as a discipline has borrowed and adapted most of its theories with the majority having been developed from the psychological and sociological disciplines (Payne, 1997; Howe, 2002; Trevithick, 2005; Teater, 2014). The *Collins Educational Dictionary of Social Work* (1995) defines theory as a 'set of propositions or hypotheses that seek to explain phenomena'. Payne (2005) takes theory to mean 'an explanation supported by evidence about why people act as they do', while Shardlow and Doel (1996) sees theory to mean 'an attempt to bring order and regularity into our experiences'.

Each of these definitions has tended to focus on a feature that has relevance in helping practitioners to develop an understanding of the term 'theory'. Howe (1987 cited in Shardlow and Doel, 1996) offers a useful way of capturing these key features by suggesting that a theory ought to enable its users to describe, to explain, to predict, to control and to bring about change to any situation. This definition of Howe's is not only useful in understanding the meaning of social work theory but also equally offers a systematic approach to address the varied presenting problems social work practitioners face on a daily basis.

Others see theory as a framework for understanding people and their situations by way of observation, description, explanation, prediction and which in turn allows practitioners to apply an intervention (Thompson, 2000; Howe, 2002; Trevithick, 2005). For Healy (2005: 95) theory acts as a guide to deciding 'who and what should be the focus of assessment and intervention' and provides varying ideas 'about the focus, objectives and processes of social work practice'.

Drawing on what seems to be a myriad of definitions, some texts have attempted to classify theories according to their level of analysis. Payne (2005) offers the following classification:

- broad-range theories offer abstract frameworks (e.g. psychoanalytic theory and systems theory);

- middle-range theories offer more specific models of intervention (e.g. cognitive behavioural theory (CBT));

- narrow-range approaches are more focused (e.g. practice wisdom).

Payne (2005) refers to Wittington and Holland (1985) and Howe (1987) to present another classification based on the perceived purposes of those who use theory:

- fixers (such as traditional social work; using existing systems to fix the problem or get the 'problem person' to fit the system);

- seekers of meaning (such as interactionists, person-centred, strengths-based, existentialist approaches);

- raisers of consciousness (such as radical social workers, radical feminists);

- revolutionaries (such as Marxist social work).

Payne (2005) proposes that theories, models and approaches serve different purposes. Theories are more abstract and offer analyses or attempts to bring about order; models tend to be more practical describing what happens in practice and offering steps to undertake structured intervention; approaches are less precisely conceptualised and allow practitioners flexibility in applying theoretical principles about particular issues or problems (Payne, 2005).

There are other detailed discussions of different types of theory in publications such as Trevithick (2005) and Teater (2014). Thompson (2010) equally addresses similar issues in his book but moves away from the traditional format of presenting theoretical approaches one after the other and focuses instead on what he perceives social workers will be likely to need to know in a range of practice situations.

To summarise this part of the discussion, it is evident that theory has a role in social work practice, although as Stepney and Ford (2000) highlight, 'theory in social work is a contested concept that is borrowed and subjected to a process of professional adaptation and refinement'.

Reflective Exercise 6.1

Think back to a client you have worked with recently. What approach did you use? Was this based on an identified theory?

Social Work Practice

There is no single straightforward procedure or guidance on how practitioners ought to apply theory in practice. Social work is practised in a range of settings (Horner, 2006). Interventions occur when professionals undertake purposeful actions based on acquired understanding and knowledge, learnt skills and their adopted values (Trevithick, 2005). Coulshed and Orme (2006: 15) offer some clarity by showing that 'knowledge gained from theory exists to inform social workers' understanding, not to dominate it'. This is supportive of the view by Healy (2005: 11) who sees theory as 'providing partial insights into direct practice within which social workers take an active role in how to apply and develop' their practice. These views are summarised well by Thompson (2010: XVI) who states that 'to do social work, is to theorise practise (to draw on sets of ideas to make sense of it) and to practise theory (to make use of those ideas in a practical context)'. Thompson (2010) takes the view that reflective practice develops from social workers' ability to theorise where they use their 'intellectual faculties and professional knowledge base to develop coherent understanding of the situations … [they] … encounter and … [their] … role within them' (XVI). What Thompson shows is that theory and practice are not separate entities but inform each other.

Others also show how practitioners draw on a range of sources to inform their practice. These include law, policy and procedures, culture and availability of resources (Muleya, 2006). Practitioners give considered attention to legal requirements, for instance the welfare checklist, when planning interventions to support children at risk or in need under the Children Act 1989 and take into account the parents' wishes on cultural norms and practices. This might be in a Children and Families Assessment Team, an Adult Safeguarding Team based in a hospital or a Contact Centre. This varied nature of the social work setting is noted by Cree (2003: 4, cited in Horner, 2006: 136) who makes an important point that social work has no essential tasks, as it 'come(s) together at a particular moment in time to frame the task … defining not just its capabilities, but also its potential'. This however does not mean social work has no purpose but

rather that social work serves a different task according to its setting and perceived presenting need.

Similarly, the definition of social work offered by the International Federation
of Social Workers (IFSW) and adopted by the International Association of Schools
of Social Work (IASSW) identifies that a practitioner draws on theory to inform
their practice. However, this definition highlights that intervention (application
of theory) occurs at the point where people interact with their environments
(IFSW, 2002). This suggests people will have capabilities to manage daily activities and social work intervention ought to be targeted to ameliorate identified
challenges at particular stages. This might entail, as Gitterman and Germain
(2008: 51) notes, interventions aimed at promoting responsive environments
that support service users' human growth, health and satisfaction in social functioning within their own environments.

Given this view of social work practice, there are a number of debates on
how practitioners accomplish essential tasks, questioning whether social work
ought to be an art or a science. Should the profession place emphasis on 'core
values' required to help and support service users or on grounded theoretical
knowledge of relevant theories of human behaviour and development?

Reflective Exercise 6.2

Based on your responses to Reflective Exercise 6.1, did you use other theories alongside your main theory? Can you justify your selection of the theories you used?

As a science, practitioners are bound by clear principles and practices, while
as an art, practitioners are more free to express their individuality and preferences. There are clear messages within literature to support the view that both
are relevant and complement each other as theory informs practice and practice
informs theory (Payne, 2005; Thompson, 2010). Milner and O'Byrne argue that
'social work's search for one cohesive theory is misplaced' and that in reality
social workers need 'a selection of practice principles and values, coupled with
a range of theoretical models and methods, as a foundation from which they
can respond creatively to the infinite range of situations they will meet' (2002:
79). This approach encourages practitioners to respond in an individualistic way
towards the service user rather than taking a 'routine approach'.

Application of Theory in Practice

Social work practitioners support people whose circumstances vary and change
depending on presenting needs, individuals' own coping capabilities and levels of

support. This creates uncertainty and depending on presenting circumstances, practitioners may undertake several assessments to clarify the issues and may need to draw on a range of different theories before deciding on the best suitable intervention. This view helps to understand the challenges practitioners face when deciding what theory to apply to inform their interventions. As noted earlier, it raises the question on what knowledge should practitioners hold and what skills should they develop to practice effectively.

Applying theory in practice raises a number of questions on how practitioners might select theory and practice methods to inform interventions. What factors might inform selection and decision making and how might practitioners use different practice methods to develop and build on service users' capacity and strengths? These questions are complex and require a detailed discussion to fully address them. Therefore, this chapter will not attempt to answer these questions, but it is important for the reader to bear these in mind in relation to the discussion that follows.

When practitioners are asked to name theories they use in their practice, the common response given is that of working 'eclectic' (Muleya, 2006). There are some, though in the minority, who can identify specific theories, models or approaches and feel able to discuss how they apply the theories, and these tend to identify middle and narrow-range theories (Muleya, 2006). These practitioners will have developed a specific way of applying a specific theory that might have led to preferred outcomes over time and they might feel reluctant to review or change their practice. For these practitioners, it might be that they no longer rely on the theory but rather on practice wisdom. This approach of applying theory may not necessarily offer opportunities to introduce new knowledge as practitioners may tend to prefer to maintain a status quo.

On the other hand, there are those practitioners who argue that they regularly apply theory in practice though are selective and only apply relevant aspects of different theories mixed up together to address presenting needs. It is this approach of applying theory that will be the focus of the remainder of this chapter.

Case Study 6.1 **Matt and Mary**

Two practitioners were chatting over lunch. Matt (Social Worker 1) describes how he was finding it difficult to evidence his work in supervision. Matt stated that he normally works through a couple of theories at the same time but is always mindful not to combine them. He stated at times the theories do not adequately address presenting issues. Mary (Social Worker 2) proudly says she adopts an approach that enables her to draw on different aspects of several theories in different combinations at the same time to address any presenting needs. Mary claims her practice enables her to evidence all her interventions and she always has good outcomes for her service users. Matt questioned the reliability and validity of Mary's approach.

What is an 'Eclectic' Approach?

In social work literature, the term is used to refer to a tendency by practitioners to draw on a wide range of theoretical understandings (Thompson, 2010). This approach does not concentrate on a single theory but rather mixes multiple theories, models, approaches, assumptions or ideas to gain a holistic overview of a particular situation which knowledge is then drawn upon to inform an intervention. This approach may seem appealing, but one needs to understand how each theory contributes to the intervention and why it is deemed relevant to be applied in the preferred manner. Here are two analogies to help illustrate 'eclectic practice' drawing on the Case Study 6.1.

Reflective Exercise 6.3

What do you see as advantages and disadvantages of Matt's approach? And of Mary's approach?

In Mary's response, there is no clear evidence of a main theory. She decides to use different theories, with the aim of combining them. Here the practitioner referring to eclecticism draws on specific aspects of different theories or models to develop an all-in-one approach that might address 'every' presented problem but with no clear awareness or understanding of how these will determine the outcome. Mary's preferred approach is uncritical as the practitioner is unaware of how each theory complements the other. As an intervention, the approach lacks clarity and coherence. Mary may draw on systems theory, strengths perspectives and task centred practice, but with no clear framework on how to apply specific aspects of these approaches. The reader is referred to Box 6.1, outlining the main characteristics of these approaches.

Box 6.1 **A brief summary of selected theoretical approaches**

General Systems Theory
Ludwig von Bertalanffy (1972) is credited for developing this theory, which he based on principles of biology. Systems theory focuses on describing how systems interact and how they are affected by actions of other systems. The theory describes how systems have the ability to grow, change and reach a steady state (Payne, 2005; Teater, 2014). It places emphasis on the importance of exchanging information and its impact on relationships. The theory differentiates between an open and closed system on the basis of how

▶

information is received and transmitted across the boundary. An open system is receptive to outside stimulus, is goal orientated, allows growth and change in order to reach or maintain a steady state, while a closed system displays none of these characteristics but tends to rely on its own energy which can lead to a breakdown when exhausted and no new energy is generated. The theory assumes systems will possess energy (Payne, 2005) or a degree of tension (Teater, 2014). In a steady state, the energy or tension is balanced and may increase as the system moves either towards or away from its goal causing it to destabilise and strive to attain a new steady state. Success will lead to a new steady state or where it is overwhelmed it might lead to system breakdown. It assumes that all organisms are systems composed of subsystems and are in turn part of a super system, and that a system can exist independently and also as part of a unit acting as a whole (Payne, 2005). The theory regards the interrelated actions of systems acting as a whole to be more complex than the sum total of what individuals bring when acting singularly, a characteristic referred to as non-summative. The theory uses a range of terms to describe interactions between systems and thereby provides practitioners with an expository framework (Payne, 2005) relevant for assessing individuals in their environment. Systems theory takes individuals, families, contexts, organisations and societies as systems and assumes there will be multiple target areas for the intervention (Teater, 2014) focused on introducing new ideas or information. A practitioner would view a service user as a system with the ability to change and reach a new steady state once provided with information. A limitation of this theory is that it does not explain what underpins and causes systems to behave, as they do not offer reasons for observed interactions. As an intervention, the theory offers practitioners descriptive tools.

Strengths Perspective

Social work literature presents the strengths-based perspective as a broad-based approach to intervention that places emphasis on individuals' strengths and capabilities moving away from the traditional focus on diagnoses and difficulties. The approach looks at positive qualities of individuals and assumes that reducing negative behaviours is dependent on building the positive side of a person's potential (Lehmann and Simmons, 2009). Strength perspective is underpinned by a number of assumptions summarised by Saleeby (2006: 15–18) into six categories and are as follows:

1 every individual, family community has strengths;

2 trauma, abuse, injury and struggle may not only be injurious but may also be sources of challenges and opportunities;

3 the upper limits of an individual's capacity to grow and change is unknown and therefore all group, individual and community aspirations should be taken seriously;

4 individuals are best served by collaborating with them;

5 each environment is full of resources;

6 care is essential to human well-being.

The intervention is relationship based and collaborative as individuals are regarded to have the inherent capacity to learn, grow and change. The role of the practitioner is that of a consultant. A limitation of this approach is its lack of emphasis on exploring deeper underlying problems and hence might not highlight risk factors and might not enable effective planning and intervention, as this is seen as unnecessary. They are more specific models of intervention developed under this perspective that address some of these limitations such as Signs of Safety and some programmes such as Strengthening Families Strengthening Communities.

Task-centred Practice

Task-centred practice has its roots in the problem-solving process developed by Perlman (1957, cited in Healy, 2005: 109) and early proponents in North America (Reid and Epstein, 1972; Reid, 1978) and later in the UK (Goldberg et al., 1985; Doel and Marsh, 1992, 2005). Task-centred practice offers a highly structured and focused way of working with service users to solve problems (Lister, 2012) of interpersonal conflict, difficulty in role performance, social transition and inadequate resources (Marsh and Doel, 2005). It assumes that service users are willing to make changes and can be assisted to identify the problems. Task-centred practice offers a structured approach with sequential steps that a practitioner follows in supporting the service users to accomplish agreed tasks which are reviewed at set intervals within a time limit. Problems are identified, rank ordered according to priority and a selected small number of the most important problems achievable within a time scale are worked through and progress is reviewed before embarking on the next set of problems. The intervention takes around 6–12 weeks. The main role of the practitioner is to motive the service user into action to accomplish set tasks through the use of deadlines (Marsh and Doel, 2005). Task-centred practice assumes the person will learn a new set of skills to draw on to address future needs. The adherence to a set structure and reliance on the abilities and willingness of service users to engage limit the usefulness of its application to interrelational and practical needs of service users with adequate skills and capacity to engage in the process.

Taking the above three theoretical approaches, when applied in Mary's preferred practice, these theories may get blurred where each method's unique characteristic features may be lost in the combination. It can be difficult to attribute the outcomes to clearly identifiable aspects of selected theories. The question arises on whether this approach is effective. This question is problematic to answer. The intervention may show some reliability (when repeated as similar outcomes emerge) but the validity (extent to which theory addresses specific problems) is much more difficult to address. Did intervention lead to outcomes?

Similarly, Matt is applying a number of approaches at the same time at different points of the intervention and, like Mary, may lack clear awareness of how each complements the other. Here Matt might be starting off from the same premise as Mary, but the difference might be that Matt draws on the unique features in a systematic manner. In practice, this may look like a kaleidoscope effect with no one dominate colour being the main theory. In this instance, some of the qualities of the theories are identifiable but the overall approach may lack coherence.

Social workers work with service users who present a range of multifaceted needs. These require careful consideration when selecting theories to assess, plan and implement interventions. As a novice or overworked (heavy caseload) practitioner, it might be tempting to adopt an eclectic approach but caution should be applied. Eclecticism does not offer a clear framework for understanding how theory informs practice and how practice informs further development of theory. It is uncritical and ideas are mixed up with no clarity and might cover up practitioners' inadequacies. This approach does not help to provide interventions that effectively empower service users or offer clear systems of accountability. Coulshed and Orme (2006) point out that in social work literature there are those who argue that selecting parts from different theories and combining them as an approach are both undisciplined and an incoherent way of working.

An Alternative Approach: Fishbone Framework for Applying Social Theory in Practice

Both students and qualified social work practitioners trying to develop an approach for applying theory in practice may initially find this to be a challenging task particularly when required to justify or defend a position involving selection and application of a specific theory. In Case Study 6.1, Mary is unable to identify with certainty and confidence of how the intervention led to perceived outcomes, while Matt might isolate the different contributions made by each intervention and argue that the outcomes are a direct result of the intervention. However, given the lack of clear systems in both examples, there is no controlled regulation over how each theory connects to the other and how they each complement the other.

A more practical approach to applying theory that addresses some of the limitations above is one that adapts the fishbone diagram (see Figure 6.1). Dr Kaoru Ishikawa, a Japanese quality control expert, is credited with inventing the fishbone diagram, also called a cause and effect diagram. The diagram is useful as a visualisation tool for categorising the potential causes of a problem in order to identify its root causes (Ishikawa, 1990).

In this chapter, I adapt this diagram to apply it to visualise and offer guidance on how social work practitioners might apply theory in practice. This might be done before undertaking the intervention, at planning stage or during the intervention. Other authors show that theories for practice are those that provide a key intellectual component of the professional base of social work (Healy, 2005: 6) and encourage practitioners to search for understanding why situations arise, why people react in certain ways and why particular interventions might be

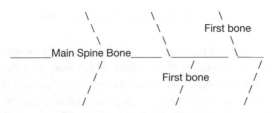

Figure 6.1 Fishbone model for applying social work theory

utilised so that theory informs practice (Coulshed and Orme, 2006: 9). As such I am not presenting this model to address these views noted by these authors.

Here I argue that the fishbone framework of applying social work theory to practice draws on the premise that a practitioner works from one main or spinal theory (bone that forms the anchor of the intervention), and where this has limitations, the practitioner draws on other theories to strengthen the planned intervention in a coordinated and coherent approach. The approach proposes an expository framework for applying theory in practice. The framework offers a transparent, practical and reliable approach that has strong validity claims.

Application: Fishbone Model

A practitioner applying the fishbone framework will work through the following stages illustrated in Figure 6.1.

Stage 1: Problem Identification (Creating the Head)

In Case Study 6.2, Mr Balls will need somewhere to stay. This might be a negotiated return home on a temporary arrangement while a long-term solution is sought, or a temporary stay with the extended family or state-funded temporary accommodation in bed and breakfast or a hostel. Mr Balls might also need support to get a job and to enable him to access health provisions.

Case Study 6.2 **Mr Balls**

Mr Balls, aged 20, lives with his parents. He has partial visual impairment in both eyes. His mother comes from a family of six siblings, who all live within walking distance of each other. Over the years, your team has supported Mr Balls and has had involvement with the extended family for various interventions.

▶

> Mr Balls contacts your office following one of his usual altercations with his parents over his unwillingness to tidy up after himself. On this occasion, the parents are very upset and have asked him to move out of their house. Mr Balls requests assistance. He informs you he would like to get a job. He is worried though about finding and registering with another GP and wants to remain with his current GP practice.

Stage 2: Identification of Main Spinal Theory

A practitioner identifies a main spinal theory to inform the intervention. Where a practitioner identifies systems theory, this will act as the main theory and therefore the anchor on which other theories will be incorporated. Systems theory will provide the practitioner with descriptive tools for understanding Mr Balls's situation, without offering a prescriptive course of action. According to Howe (1990: 52), systems theory is 'interested in the orderly relationships that exist between people … the nature of such order, how it comes about and how it is maintained' (see Box 6.1). This reflects the philosophy of social work as its concern with people's social connections and relationships (Payne, 2005).

Systems theory will enable the social worker to make note of the different systems that Mr Balls interacts with and the interaction between these systems. This scenario highlights: a network of people, families and agencies; the breakdown of stability within the main family; and the need to re-establish relationships within this family as well as establishing new relationships with other agencies. Systems theory will offer awareness on what new connections need to be established but will not prescribe specific actions to be undertaken. It promotes a holistic perspective, enabling the practitioner to gain an overview of such complex networks and gain an understanding of the influences of numerous factors on Mr Balls and his situation.

In this fishbone framework, the practitioner has flexibility to select other theories that address aspects of the presenting needs that systems theory might not highlight. In our illustration, there is a need to encourage Mr Balls to accomplish certain tasks within an agreed time scale. This leads to the next stage of this model.

Stage 3: Identification of First Bone (Secondary) Approaches

Systems theory would have the capacity to highlight existence of different relationships and the nature of the flow of information (input) but would not necessarily prescribe how to get Mr Balls to accomplish the desired outcomes within a timescale. In this regard, task-centred practice with the capacity to achieve this can be used to specifically address this need; thus, task-centred practice will complement systems theory, the main spinal intervention.

In the fishbone diagram, task-centred practice is then connected to the spine, as one of the first bones (secondary theories) with clear annotation stating how and what will be addressed. Strengths perspectives may be added as another first bone (secondary theory) aimed at providing practice guidance on aspects of the intervention aimed at developing Mr Balls's own coping mechanisms. Where need arises, other second bones would be added to the spine of the first bones, and so forth.

In this illustration, task-centred practice is applied as an effective intervention aimed at addressing limitations in systems theory's assumption and failure to address social order. Systems theory assumes that everything fits neatly into a social order, and in order to maintain such stability, there is a need and preparedness to regulate and control behaviour (Payne, 2005). Therefore, the practitioner retains power and makes the decisions. Trevithick (2005: 268) quotes Rogers's argument that for people to move forward 'they need a non-directive stance, where their thoughts, feelings and actions are not subject to advice, interpretation, criticism, confrontation or challenge beyond encouraging people to clarify what they see to be happening'. Howe (1990. p, 54) states that through the analysis of a system, the practitioner can determine the area of the current 'imbalance' and therefore where to target change to create a new equilibrium. This would suggest that it is the practitioner who decides what the issues and problems are based on a pre-determined idea of what is acceptable social order (White, 2008). To address these limitations, and empower Mr Balls, a practitioner will need to draw on other theories.

The practitioner may draw on task-centred practice to address these concerns of oppressive practice, under the fishbone framework, applying the approach to target limitations of systems theory whilst maintaining the theory as the main spinal approach. In applying task-centred practice, a practitioner will take the aims identified by Mr Balls as the starting point for planning these aspects of his needs thereby empowering him to make informed decisions. In contrast, the worker informed by systems theory may be less likely to take the goals described by Mr Balls as the starting point. Instead, their analysis of the wider system and the context in which Mr Balls exists may lead to over-complication and redirection. Therefore, the first bones are needed to complement what already exists. However, the additional theories (first bones) do not lose their qualities, as the practitioner would implement task-centred practice alongside a systems approach.

Stage 4: Identification of Other Additional Approaches

The model allows practitioners to continually add new approaches as and when new needs arise, acknowledging that human nature is complex and problems people face are complex and fluid. Throughout this process, the practitioner remains mindful of the aim of the first bones (secondary) theories being to complement the main spinal theory. This visualisation may enable practitioners to develop better awareness of a planned intervention (or as it develops), its strengths and limitations when applied as proposed. The fishbone framework offers a stronger basis to argue for reliability and validity, and opportunities to engage in both reflection and reflexivity.

Social work literature (Trevithick, 2005; Thompson, 2010) cautions that applying theory to practice can involve complex analyses beyond simplistic clear connections between theory and practice. The range of theoretical approaches act as guides to deciding 'who and what should be the focus of assessment and intervention' and provides varying ideas 'about the focus, objectives and processes of social work practice' (Healy, 2005: 95). The focus of an intervention may concentrate upon different individuals and groups and might take several forms depending upon their purpose (Trevithick, 2005). Therefore, this model is presented as an alternative approach to guide practitioners in their quest to apply theory in practice rather than as an intervention method in itself.

Reflective Exercise 6.4

What other theories or models might a practitioner working with Mr Balls draw on?

Conclusion

This chapter has addressed the challenges of applying theory in practice. This discussion has proposed an alternative approach for applying theoretical knowledge in practice that maintains the key features (principles) of selected theories whilst equally allowing practitioners to address the approach's limitations by systematically introducing other theories to maximise its effectiveness and offer better outcomes for service users. The chapter has presented this framework as one that can be applied by professionals at all the three levels of capability (prequalifying, qualified Social Worker/Experienced Social Worker and Advanced Level) identified under the Professional Capabilities Framework (PCF).

Progress Check

Practitioners need to understand both their work environments and that of service users in order to select the relevant theory to inform their practice. The discussion in the section 'What Is an "Eclectic" Approach?' and the case studies illustrate the benefits of critical understanding of how a theory is applied in practice. This requires capabilities within

▶

all the domains of the PCF at all the three levels of capability (pre-qualifying, qualified Social Worker/Experienced Social Worker and Advanced Level). However, two domains – 'knowledge' and 'intervention and skills' – underpin these capabilities as stated:

1 Under Knowledge:

Demonstrate a critical understanding of the application to social work of research, theory and knowledge from sociology, social policy, psychology and health (5.1).

2 Under Intervention and Skills:

Select and use appropriate frameworks to assess, give meaning to, plan, implement and review effective interventions and evaluate the outcomes, in partnership with service users (7.5).

Use a planned and structured approach, informed by social work methods, models and tools, to promote positive change and independence to prevent harm (7.6).

These are further highlighted in skills embedded within the Health and Care Professions Council's Standards of Proficiency for Social Workers in England (HCPC, 2012), for example as: 'be able to draw on appropriate knowledge and skills to inform practice' (SoPs 14).

Chapter Summary

This chapter proposes a framework for applying theoretical knowledge in practice that focuses on a principal theory and, whilst maintaining its key features (principles), incorporates other secondary theories. It is argued that practitioners so often lack clear awareness and clarity of how their efforts at combining different theories lead to observed outcomes. The proposed expository framework draws on the fishbone model and allows practitioners to address a selected principal theory's limitations systematically by drawing on other theories to maximise its effectiveness and assess clear outcomes for service users.

Further Reading

- Coulshed, V., and Orme, J., (2006) *Social Work Practice*, 4th edition. Basingstoke: Palgrave Macmillan.

- Teater, B. (2014) *An Introduction to Applying Social Work Theories and Methods*. Berkshire: Open University Press

- Trevithick, P. (2005) *Social Work Skills: A Practice Handbook*, 2nd edition. Berkshire: Open University Press.

References

Bertalanffy, L. von., (1972) The History and Status of General Systems Theory. In Klier, G. (ed.), *Trends in General Systems Theory*, New York: Wiley, 21–41

Coulshed, V., and Orme, J., (2006) *Social Work Practice*, 4th Edition. Basingstoke: Palgrave Macmillan

Doel, M. (2002) Task Centred Practice. In Adams, R., Dominelli, L. and Payne, M. (eds.), *Social Work: Themes Issues and Critical Debates*. Basingstoke: Macmillan, 191–6

Gitterman, A., and Germain, C., (2008) *The Life Model of Social Work Practice Advances in Theory and Practice*. 3rd revised edition. New York: Columbia University Press.

Goldberg, E. M., Gibbons, J. and Sinclair, I. (1985) *Problems, Tasks and Outcomes*. London: George, Allen and Unwin

Health and Care Professions Council (2012) Standards of Proficiency for Social Workers in England. Publication code: 20120521POLPUB

Healy, K. (2005) *Social Work Theories in Context: Creating Frameworks for Practice*. Basingstoke: Palgrave Macmillan

Horner, N., (2006) *What is Social Work: Contexts and Perspectives,* 2nd edition. Basingstoke: Learning Matters

Howe, D., (1987) *An Introduction to Social Work Theory,* Aldershot: Wildwood House Ltd International Federation of Social Workers (IFSW) (2002) *Definition of Social Work*. Berne, Switzerland: IFSW.

Howe, D., (1990) *An Introduction to Social Work Theory*. Aldershot: Ashgate Publishing

Howe, D. (2002) Relating Theory to Practice. In Davies, M. (ed.), *The Blackwell Companion to Social Work*, 2nd edition. Oxford: Blackwell.

Ishikawa, K. (1990) *Introduction to Quality Control*. J. H. Loftus (trans.). Tokyo: 3A Corporation

Lehmann, P., and Simmons, C., (eds) (2009) Strengths-based Batterer Intervention: A New Paradigm in Ending Family Violence. New York: Springer

Lister, P., (2012) *Integrating Social Work Theory and Practice: A Practical Skills Guide*. Oxford: Routledge.

Marsh, P., and Doel, M., (1992) *Task-Centred Social Work*, Farnham: Ashgate

Marsh, P., and Doel, M., (2005) *The Task-Centred Book*, London: Routledge/Community Care.

Milner, J. and O'Byrne, P. (2002) *Assessment in Social Work*, 2nd edition. Basingstoke: Palgrave Macmillan.

Muleya, W. (2006) A Comparative Study of Social Work in Context in Zambia and England, *International Social Work*, 49 (4): 445–457.

Payne, M. (1997) *Modern Social Work Theory*. Basingstoke: Palgrave Macmillan.

Payne, M. (2005) *Modern Social Work Theory*, 3rd edition. Basingstoke: Palgrave Macmillan.

Reid, W. J. (1972) *The Task-Centred Casework*. New York: Columbia University Press.

Reid, W. J. (1978) *The Task-Centred System*. New York: Columbia University Press.

Saleeby, D. (2006) *Strengths Perspective in Social Work Practice*, 5th edition. Boston: Pearson/Allyn & Bacon.

Shardlow, S. and Doel, M. (1996) *Practice Learning and Teaching*. London: Macmillan.

Stepney P. and Ford, D. (2000) *Social Work Models, Methods and Theories: A Framework for Practice*. Lyme Regis: Russell House Publishing.

Teater, B. (2014) An Introduction to Applying Social Work Theories and Methods. Berkshire: Open University Press

Thomas. M., and Pierson, J., (1995) Collins Educational Dictionary of Social Work. Hammersmith: Collins Educational.

Thompson, N. (2000). *Theory and Practice in Human Services*. Maidenhead: Open University Press.

Thompson, N. (2010) *Theorizing Social Work Practice*. Basingstoke: Palgrave Macmillan.

Trevithick, P. (2005) *Social Work Skills: A Practice Handbook*, 2nd edition. Berkshire: Open University Press.

White, J. (2008). Family Therapy. In Davies, M. (ed.), *The Blackwell Companion to Social Work*, 3rd edition. Oxford: Blackwell.

Whittington, C., and Holland. R., (1985) A Framework for Theory in Social Work *Issues in Social Work Education*, 5(1).

7

LEGAL SKILLS FOR SOCIAL WORKERS

Susan Watson

Introduction

Social workers are subject to, empowered, constrained and guided by law. They are expected to understand the law that is relevant to their social work practice which includes recognition of how the law can both promote and deny rights to service users. This chapter provides a straightforward explanation of why legal knowledge is vital for social workers and students and how legal skills can promote good practice and enable empowerment of service users. It will also recognise that for a significant proportion of service users, the law can operate to limit their rights and disempower them. The chapter identifies different legal sources and key areas of knowledge applicable to all social work practice. It uses case studies to demonstrate how important legal knowledge and skills are in social work practice. It should be read in conjunction with the Health and Care Professions Council's (HCPC) Standards of Proficiency for Social Workers in England (HCPC, 2012) and the College of Social Work's Professional Capabilities Framework (The College of Social Work, 2012) which identify the legal skills and knowledge that social workers are required to have to qualify and enter practice.

Why Are Law and Legal Skills Important to Social Workers?

The title of 'social worker' is protected by law and only those registered with the HCPC can use this title (s. 61 Care Standards Act 2000). Social workers, as well as being social care professionals, are creations of statute (Local Authority and Social Services Act 1970). Brayne et al. (2015) describe social workers as 'agents of statutory control' (51). They must work within the law and can be held accountable for what they do.

Neither students nor social workers can be expected to know all the laws that are relevant to social work practice but it is helpful to be familiar with law that affects the service users they work with and they should have a good working knowledge of the key areas of law that determine how they carry out their role. In short, they should be aware of what duties the law places upon them and what power the law gives them. Brayne et al. (2015) note how this distinction determines social work priorities. If the law places a duty on social workers, then they must carry out this duty, as a matter of priority. Added to this, a service user may take legal action if they are unhappy about how this duty has been carried out. A successful legal action against the local authority and/or the individual social worker is unlikely if the local authority or social worker is acting properly under a power. Apart from the law that governs the specialist area of their practice, for example, work with children and families or adult social care, social workers should be aware of the requirements of human rights legislation (Human Rights Act 1998) and equality law (Equality Act 2010), which are discussed below.

The legal skills that social workers are expected to acquire are those of understanding the effect of the law, knowing how a particular law is likely to apply in practice and developing the ability to keep themselves updated with law which can be subject to rapid change. To keep themselves updated, students and social workers should keep an eye out for changes in the law via the news, in Community Care, via online updates from practitioners' websites or by attending legal updates organised for lawyers and social workers.

As Johns (2011) notes, the law cannot provide guidance for a social worker in every situation. It does, however, provide a framework for decision making and, if used effectively, can be a way to ensure that the rights of service users are respected.

What is Law?

Law can be described as a set of rules which come from defined sources. A discussion of all the sources of law is beyond the scope of this chapter, but see Brammer (2015) and Brayne et al. (2015) for a fuller discussion of the different sources of law.

1 Acts of Parliament
Acts of Parliament or primary legislation are also called statutes and, for social workers, they are the most important sources of law. Almost all of social work practice is affected by statute and may also be changed by statute. Some examples of statutes are as follows:

The Children Act 1989

The Human Rights Act 1998

The Equality Act 2010

The Children and Families Act 2014

Statute may place duties on local authorities which require them to provide services to defined groups of service users.

---

s.17 (1) The Children Act 1989:

It shall be the general duty of every local authority (in addition to the other duties imposed upon them by this part):

(a) to safeguard and promote the welfare of children within their area who are in need; and

(b) so far as is consistent with that duty, to promote their upbringing of such children by their families, by providing a range and level of services appropriate to those children's needs.

Local authorities have a range of duties to all children in the area who are 'in need' and the power to provide services for them and their families. The statute also provides a definition of who children in need are:

---

s.17 (10) The Children Act 1989:

(a) he is unlikely to achieve or maintain a reasonable standard of health or development without appropriate provision for him of services by a local authority under this Part;

(b) his health and development is likely to be significantly impaired, without the provision for him of services by a local authority; or

(c) he is disabled.

In addition to the general duty owed to children 'in need', Part 1 Schedule 2 to the Act contains a number of specific duties to provide for the families of children 'in need', for example provision of services for disabled children and their families.

2 Delegated legislation
A number of statutes have powers within them that enable an individual, usually the Secretary of State or an organisation like a local authority, to make delegated legislation which has the full force of the law. Delegated legislation takes many forms, including statutory instruments, laws and regulations.

3 Regulations
Regulations often provide the detail that adds to the duty or power within the Act of Parliament or primary legislation. An example of this is The Breaks for

Carers of Disabled Children Regulations 2011 which gives more detail about how the local authority should perform their duties to provide for carers (including considering their needs) and what types of services it would be reasonably practicable to offer them (such as day care or overnight care).

4 Guidance
Formal policy guidance is identified as being issued under statue. As an example, Working Together to Safeguard Children (Department of Education, 2015) is issued under the Local Authority Social Services Act 1970 s.7 and the Children Act 2004 s.10, 11, 14B and 16. This guidance must be followed and if it is departed from, without good reason, it is considered to be a breach of the law (R v Islington Borough Council, ex parte Rixon [1997] ELR 66).

5 The common law: case law
The common law is made up of decisions about particular matters brought before the court which is called case law. Case law is developed on the basis of precedent which means that certain laws are applied to a particular set of facts. When a case with a new set of facts is considered by the court, it is expected that where the facts are similar to a previous decision, the court will reach a similar decision to one that it reached earlier. Precedent can be created by:

Developing the common law, or;

By interpreting statutes. This happens where the court rules on the meaning of the words in a particular statute. This then creates a precedent on the interpretation of that statutory provision which has to be followed by courts lower down the system and by anyone affected by that provision.

For example, in X Council v B (Emergency Protection Orders) [2004] EWHC 2015 (Fam), the court gave guidance on the use of the Emergency Protection Order (EPO) under s.44 Children Act 1989. An EPO is used to remove a child from their parents on an emergency basis; it is a power that the court will grant to the social worker when there is reasonable cause to believe that the child is suffering or likely to suffer significant harm. The local authority in that case had obtained EPOs, lasting eight days, without telling the mother, and the children were taken into foster care. The judge, Mr Justice Munby, was concerned that these EPOs had lasted for more than 24–48 hours and made it clear that there is a requirement of 'necessity' and 'imminent danger' to justify the removal of a child from their parents on an emergency basis without informing the parents first. Following this case, in Re X (Emergency Protection Orders) [2006] EWHC 510, Mr Justice McFarlane agreed with Mr Justice Munby's guidance and stated that this guidance should be made available to all lower courts hearing an application for an EPO. The applicant authority was charged with the responsibility for providing this guidance to the court.

Human Rights Law

'Human rights are for everyone,' Baroness Hale said recently in the case of P (by his litigation friend the Official Solicitor) (Appellant) v Cheshire West and Chester Council and another (Respondents) [2014] UKSC 19. The point that she was making, in a case where the court was required to decide whether severely disabled people were being deprived of their liberty, was a pertinent one for social workers. She reminds us that social workers must practise in a way that respects the human rights of all service users and should take particular care where they are vulnerable and perhaps even more susceptible to breaches of their human rights. In the course of their duties, social workers are required to make difficult decisions. A key legal skill involves balancing competing rights of service users, weighing the rights of one person against another or weighing a person's rights against the interests of the community. The Human Rights Act 1998 (HRA) has had a significant influence on the development of the law, and areas of social work practice have been challenged by the Act. It is, therefore, important that social workers have a good working knowledge of how the framework of the Act operates.

The HRA was drafted to give effect to the rights and freedoms under the European Convention on Human Rights (1950). Britain has been a signatory to this since 1951, yet, until the Human Rights Act 1998 came into force, its provisions were not enforceable under the domestic law of this country. People who complained that their rights had been breached could take a case to the European Court of Human Rights (ECtHR); this was a slow and expensive process, taking five years or longer. The HRA now enables a claim which alleges a breach of the Convention to be heard in the English courts. People can still take a claim to the ECtHR but only after the matter has been dealt with in the British courts. The courts are now obliged:

- to decide all cases brought before them compatibly with Convention law (s.6(1)(2) (3));

- to interpret existing and future legislation compatibly with the Convention (s.3);

- to take into account relevant case law from the ECtHR (s.2 (1)).

Public Authorities

The Act requires public authorities to carry out their functions in accordance with Convention rights and makes it unlawful to act in a way that is not compatible with those rights (s.6(1) HRA, 1998). Public authorities include any person whose functions are of a public nature (s.6(3)). This means that local authorities and the social workers, who are employed by them, must act in a way that

promotes the rights protected by the HRA. This applies not only to social workers but also includes police, health authorities and private providers of care who
are exercising functions of a public nature. This can be problematic for those
service users who receive care from a private provider.

YL v Birmingham City Council [2007] UKHL 27

YL was an 84-year-old woman with Alzheimer's who lived in a private care home. She
faced eviction because of her family's difficult behaviour on visits. Were she to be moved,
medical opinion said she would be placed at risk. It was argued by her lawyers that if she
were to be evicted that her right to respect for family life would be breached. The issue
was whether the care home was exercising functions of a public nature because the
local authority funded her placement. The House of Lords decided that the care home
was not a public authority. It was simply carrying out a 'socially useful business for profit'
(Lord Scott). Just because some of its residents were publicly funded did not change its
private character.

In effect, the private providers of care were not required to act compatibly
with the HRA, so service users in this position were not protected by the HRA.
Fortunately, the concerning and limiting effects of this decision were reversed
by the enactment of s.145 Health and Social Care Act 2008 which ensures that
people who receive publicly funded care in the private sector have the protection of the HRA.

Convention Rights

The HRA is found at http://www.legislation.gov.uk/ukpga/1998/42/contents,
and the Convention rights are in Schedule one of the Act. It is beyond the scope
of this chapter to consider all the rights in detail, so the focus will be on some
key rights, which most often impact on social work practice.

Article 2 establishes a right to life. This right is limited in clearly defined circumstances which include the use of force to prevent unlawful violence. Brayne
et al. (2015) suggest that this right might be relevant to a local authority social
services department where there is a failure to act to prevent the death of a child
at the hands of their parents. Whilst there are numerous examples of these
tragedies, no such action has yet been taken against a local authority in England
and Wales.

Article 3 is the right not to be subjected to torture or to inhumane or degrading treatment or punishment; this is an absolute right without limitation or
qualification. This is relevant to social workers in respect of their duties to protect
people from abuse. In the case of Z and others v UK (Application No 29392/95)

(2001) 34 EHRR 97, the ECtHR awarded damages to children against the local authority that had failed to remove them from home over a period of over four years, when they had suffered both physical and emotional abuse. This abuse reached the threshold of Article 3 and the local authority had breached the children's Convention rights because they had failed to take action.

Article 5 is the right not to be deprived of liberty and security meaning that a person can only be detained if the procedure has been carried out lawfully and the person detained must be able to challenge this detention in a timely manner. In HL v UK [2005] 40 EHRR 32, the UK was held by the ECtHR to have breached Article 5 because there was a lack of procedural protection available to patients, lacking capacity, who were detained informally in residential care settings. The common law principle of acting in the patients 'best interests' did not include sufficient procedural safeguards.

Article 6 provides for the right to a fair and public hearing within a reasonable time by an independent and impartial tribunal established by law. This article is not only relevant to court proceedings but also to how decisions are made by social workers in child Protection Conferences and how social workers use their statutory powers.

Article 8 is the right to respect for private and family life; any interference with this must be lawful, necessary and proportionate. This right is a qualified right so it is permissible to interfere in family life. The following case study example, Josh, shows how a social worker may justify drastic interference in a family's life.

Case Study 7.1 **Josh**

Josh is a five-year-old boy who lives with his mother and father. His parents have long-standing difficulties with substance misuse, and Josh has been subject to both physical and emotional abuse. At a multi-agency child protection Conference, it is decided that the services and this support have been provided to support Josh living with his family are no longer working because he continues to suffer significant harm. It is decided that a care order should be sought to enable him to be placed in local authority foster care.

The legal framework for social work with children and families allows for the use of compulsory powers, under the Children Act 1989, where other support fails. If the decision to compulsorily remove Josh from his family is carried out by the proper use of statutory powers, most likely through the application for a care order, then the local authority will have acted lawfully. The decision to remove Josh must also be seen as necessary and this decision will be made by the court considering, firstly, whether he is suffering or likely to suffer harm and, secondly, whether it is in his best interests to be placed in the care of the local authority (s.31 Children Act 1989). Finally, the decision to remove Josh from his parents must be seen as proportionate; there is no need to use a sledgehammer to crack a nut. What this means is that the aim of safeguarding Josh from harm could not have been achieved through any less drastic action taken by the local authority. A local authority is expected to offer a reasonable level of support to Josh and his family to enable him to remain with them. If the local authority has fulfilled its duties in relation to the support offered to Josh and his family, and which has not worked, then a decision to remove him from his parents by the court is unlikely to be seen as disproportionate.

Equality Law

The PCF 3.2 enjoins social workers, with reference to current legislative requirements, to recognise personal and organisational discrimination and oppression and with guidance make use of a range of approaches to challenge them. Knowledge of the extent to which the law can contribute to the prevention of discrimination, promote equality of opportunity and its limitations in doing so is of crucial importance.

Article 14 of the ECHR prohibits discrimination. This is not, however, a free standing right. Article 14 provides that the Convention rights are to be enjoyed without discrimination on grounds such as sex, race, colour, language, religion, political or other opinion, national or social origin, association with a national minority, property, birth or other status. The ECHR, therefore, impacts where enjoyment of the rights under the Convention is prevented because of discrimination.

The Equality Act 2006 established the Equality and Human Rights Commission (EHRC) and placed a duty upon it, under s.3, to support and encourage a society where:

- people's ability to achieve their potential is not limited by prejudice or discrimination;
- there is respect for, and protection of, each individual's human rights;
- there is respect for the dignity and worth of each individual;
- each individual has an equal opportunity to participate in society;
- there is mutual respect between groups based on understanding and valuing of diversity and on shared respect for equality and human rights.

The establishment of the EHRC was the first stage in developing one framework to promote equality in the UK. Since then the Equality Act 2010 has consolidated and replaced the previous discrimination legislation. It has three main effects which are as follow:

1. *Prohibits conduct towards those with protected characteristics.* It is unlawful to discriminate against a person with one of the 'protected characteristics': age, disability, gender reassignment, marriage and civil partnership, pregnancy and maternity, race, religion or belief, sex and sexual orientation (s.4) by acting in a prohibited way through direct discrimination (s.13), indirect discrimination (s.19), discrimination arising from disability (s.15), failure to make reasonable adjustments for a disability (s.21), harassment (s.26) or victimisation (s.27). The act also makes it unlawful to discriminate against people in the provision of services (s.29); this applies to all the protected characteristics except age in relation to people under 18 and marriage/civil partnership (s.28 (1)).

2. *Places a general equality duty on public bodies.* The equality duty places three aims on public bodies: to take steps to eliminate prohibited conduct, promote equality of treatment and foster good relations between different groups of people (s.149). Promoting equality of treatment means that public bodies are also required to remove or minimise disadvantage, take steps to meet need and encourage people to participate in public life (s.149 (3)).

3. *Allows for positive action.* This enables public bodies to take positive action (in defined circumstances) to support inclusion of people with protected characteristics (s.158).

What Are the Implications for Social Work Practice?

It is important to note that the Act places an emphasis on an individual person to make a claim of discrimination; this is most likely to occur in the employment context; enforcement of the Act relies largely on individual action rather than enforcement by the EHRC. The EHRC website http://www.equalityhumanrights. com/ offers advice to individuals who wish to pursue a complaint of discrimination. However, where there has been discrimination in the provision of services, the implications for social work practice are obvious. Examples of this might be failing to arrange an accessible meeting place for a physically disabled service user or not providing an interpreter for a service user who could not speak English and who would not be able to effectively participate in a meeting without someone to interpret for them.

An individual with a particular protected characteristic is entitled to expect a service on the same terms as someone else without that characteristic; a complaint which received a considerable amount of media attention was the case of Bull and another (Appellants) v Hall and another (Respondents) [2013] UKSC 73. Mr Preddy and Mr Hall, who were civil partners, were refused a double bedded room at the bed and breakfast run by Mr and Mrs Bull. Mr and Mrs Bull believed that sexual relations outside heterosexual marriage were sinful and so were not prepared to offer Mr Preddy and Mr Hall a double bed although they were prepared to offer them a twin-bedded room or a single room. The Supreme Court held that the actions of Mr and Mrs Bull were unlawful under equality legislation and that this was not a breach of their Article 9 rights of freedom of thought, conscience and religion. To put this into context, a service user may complain of being denied a service because they are gay or from an ethnic minority, and social workers should consider what steps they could take to advocate for and support the service user in dealing with this breach of the law.

The EHRC website gives case examples of how the equality duty can be carried out: in the case of the Gypsy and travelling community, work has been undertaken to develop positive relationships with this community which reduces negative press coverage and promotes the positive identity and heritage of the community (http://www.equalityhumanrights.com/about-us/our-work/key-projects/good-relations/gypsies-and-travellers-simple-solutions-for-living-together).

Finally, the influence of the Equality Act 2010 on social work practice is vividly evidenced in the case of Re C (A Child) [2014] EWCA Civ 128:

C, who was 17 months old at the time of the appeal, had been accommodated by the local authority in foster care when she was six days old with the consent of her parents. Her mother has learning disabilities, including a speech and hearing impairment, and her father is profoundly deaf and communicates using British Sign Language. When her parents withdrew their consent to her accommodation two weeks later, the local authority initiated care proceedings, and C has been in foster care since then. At the final hearing, the Judge decided that it was not in C's best interests to remain with her parents, and he made a care order and a placement order for C's adoption. When her parents appealed against this decision, the Court of Appeal was critical of the lower court, the local authority and the Child and Family Court Advisory Service (CAFCASS) and found that there had been a lack of proper provision (an interpreter from the deaf community) to enable C's father to take part in the court proceedings and local authority assessment. In setting aside the care order and placement order and substituting this for an interim care order, Lord Justice McFarlane said:

'The court as an organ of the state, the local authority and CAFCASS must all function now within the terms of the Equality Act 2010. It is simply not an option to fail to afford the right level of regard to an individual who has these unfortunate disabilities' (para. 26).

Information Sharing, Record Keeping and the Law

Social workers gather and process a huge amount of sensitive and personal information in relation to the service users they work with. The law provides a framework to protect individuals from the misuse of this information and social workers need to know how this applies to them. There is an immediate tension in this area. It is important to both share information to protect service users and maintain the trust of service users when they have provided information in confidence. Here the law plays an important part in balancing competing interests some of which are listed below:

- To what extent do social workers have rights to obtain information?

- Can social workers protect the sources of information they obtain?

- What are the limits placed on social workers about the information that can be obtained?

- When are social workers obliged to share this information, even when it was obtained in confidence?

- How secure are records created by social workers from access by others?

- What rights do clients or the public have to gain access to records created by social workers?

From a rights perspective Article 10 HRA is the right to freedom of expression (or free speech), which includes the right to receive and impart information. It is, however, a qualified right and interference is permitted as necessary in the interests of individuals and the community. Article 8 contains the right to privacy in family life. Information sharing may cause these articles to come directly into conflict if information, which has been obtained in confidence from a service user, is required to be shared with another person or agency. There is a clear tension between the competing demands of confidentiality and access to information. It is important to note that whilst social workers are under a duty of confidentiality to service users, there are instances where it is permissible to disclose confidential information. Disclosure is permitted where there are safeguarding concerns about a child or vulnerable adult (DFE 2015).

In order to assist practitioners in making a professional judgement, the government has produced guidance – Information Sharing: Advice for Practitioners Providing Safeguarding Services to Children, Young People Parents and Carers (DFE 2015) – to support good practice on legal and professional information sharing. Of particular note is that the guidance is intended to prevent a need from becoming more acute and difficult to meet. At the other end of the spectrum it could be the difference between life and death (1).

In deciding to share information, the guidance sets out questions that should be answered and further information on how to answer these questions (10–12).

Inevitably, however, this will be a decision for your professional judgement with reference to the legal and policy frameworks that guide your practice. With this in mind, it is important to consider the requirements of the Data Protection Act 1998 which regulates the holding of information by public authorities. This requires people or organisations that hold personal information, termed as data controllers in the Act, to register with the Information Commissioner, and enables people, whose personal information is held, to access that information. At the heart of the Act are the data protection principles (Schedule 1) which lay down the required standards applicable to holding and using personal data. Brayne et al. (2015) provide a useful explanation of how these principles operate in the context of Social work practice (126).

Access by Service Users to Personal Information

A service user has the right to access personal information held about them (ss.7–9 Data Protection Act 1998) by writing to the data controller with a subject access request; this data must be made available unless it is exempt. Information can also be withheld if disclosure of it would cause serious harm to a service user or other person's health, including that of a professional. Service users can see only their records. Information provided by a child that they did not expect to be shown to their parents would be exempt. Brayne et al. (2015) note that this means that a parent accused of abusing their child would be unlikely to be given access to their child's records. If this information had been recorded on the parent's file, then the parent would also be unlikely to be allowed to see this if it was given, by the child, in the expectation of the parent not being given access to it.

If the social work file contains confidential information about a service user and the local authority is asked by a third party to disclose that information so that it can be used as evidence in court then, unless the service user consents, the local authority has a duty to assert public interest immunity. This means that the local authority may refuse to disclose information in a court case where a child has given them information that they have been abused because of the public interest in maintaining the confidentiality of information given to the authorities responsible for protecting children from abuse. Public immunity is not absolute, however, and must be balanced against the public interest in a fair trial. The court can order disclosure to the extent necessary for there to be a fair hearing even if that creates difficulties for, or distress to, the service user who gave the information in confidence to the local authority. The case of Re A (A Child) [2012] UKSC 60 demonstrates the difficulties of balancing Article 3 (right not to suffer inhuman or degrading treatment), Article 8 (right to respect for private and family life) and Article 6 (right to a fair trial).

The Supreme Court summarised the issues as follows:

> We are asked in this case to reconcile the irreconcilable. On the one hand, there is the interest of a vulnerable young woman (X) who made an allegation in confidence to the authorities that while she was a child she had been seriously sexually abused by the father of a little girl (A) who is now aged 10. On the other hand we have the interests of that little girl, her mother and her father, in having that allegation properly investigated and tested. These interests are not only private to the people involved. There are also public interests, on the one hand, in maintaining the confidentiality of this kind of communication, and, on the other, in the fair and open conduct of legal disputes. On both sides there is a public interest in protecting both children and vulnerable young adults from the risk of harm. (para. 1)

The court concluded that 'X's privacy rights are not a sufficient justification for the grave compromise of the fair trial and family life rights of the parties which non-disclosure would entail' [para. 35].

Using the Law and Legal Skills

Consider the following case study, Amelia, and ask yourself the following questions as you do.

- What legal knowledge does a social worker need in this situation and what legal sources should they consult to ensure that they have the correct knowledge to deal with this situation?

- What needs to be considered when weighing up the competing interests and rights in this situation?

- To what extent does the law assist in preventing discrimination and promoting equality?

Case study 7.2 **Amelia**

Amelia (aged 23 months) lives with her mother, Jen, and father Kamel. Jen has learning disabilities and is hearing impaired, she finds it difficult to communicate with people she is unfamiliar with and her comprehension is badly affected when she is in stressful situations. Kamel's first language is Arabic and he has a limited use of English. Social services become involved with the family when they receive a referral from the health visitor who is very concerned about Amelia. Amelia had not attended any developmental

▶

checks, and when the health visitor visited the family home she observed that Amelia was not able to bear her own weight and could only move slowly by holding onto the sofa. Additionally, Jen told the health visitor that Amelia rarely ate solid food because she was a fussy eater and would only drink milk from a bottle. There was also a large amount of bruising on her legs. During the health visitor's visit, Kamel returned and insisted that the health visitor leave. He said there was nothing wrong with Amelia. She was just 'slow' like her mother and that he didn't want the family to be interfered with.

Relevant Factual Issues

Students and social workers will easily identify the relevant factual issues raised by this case study and that is the starting point in identifying how the law empowers them to intervene and places a duty upon them to act. The key factual issues raised by this scenario include the following:

- harm to Amelia: her failure to meet developmental milestones needs further investigation, and the considerable bruising on her legs;

- the parenting skills of Jane and Kamel who show limited understanding of Amelia's needs;

- potential communication difficulties with Jane and Kamel.

Identification of the Law

Social workers should begin by understanding where their power and duty to act comes from. And then they should consult any guidance attached to that statutory authority. Case law will also provide guidance about how the statute is to be interpreted. Here, intervention in respect of Amelia is governed by the Children Act 1989, and social workers should consult Working Together to Safeguard Children (2015) for guidance on how a social worker should approach this type of referral. The guidance both advises and demonstrates, using flow charts, the expected action that should be taken in relation to the type of intervention that the referral suggests. The questions for the local authority social worker are whether Amelia requires immediate protection and whether the local authority should take urgent action by applying for an Emergency Protection Order (s.44 CA 1989), whether she is a child in need and should be assessed under (s.17 CA 1989) or whether there is reasonable cause to suspect that Amelia is suffering or is likely to suffer significant harm (s.47 CA 1989) and should be assessed under this section. The local authority will determine what services should be offered to the family and what further specialist assessments are necessary.

The assessment carried out by the local authority should be timely and comply with local protocols for assessment. The facts of the case study suggest that there is reasonable cause to suspect that Amelia is suffering harm. Thus a social worker would conduct an assessment under s.47. Other partners of the local authority such as housing and health are required to cooperate with local authority social services to enable the social worker to complete a full assessment (s.27 CA 1989). A decision about whether a child is suffering present harm and/or will suffer future harm is made by the social worker in conjunction with other professionals involved with the child. Harm includes ill-treatment or impaired health and development and harm caused by seeing or hearing the ill-treatment of another (s.31(9)). This is particularly relevant in Amelia's case because it embraces possible impairment to her development as a result of poor parenting as well as physical injury. The age and development of the child is important as Amelia's development should be compared with a similar child (s.31 (10)). Notably the harm must be significant, which has been interpreted by the court to mean considerable or noteworthy or important (Re MA (Children) (Care Proceedings: Threshold Criteria) [2009] EWCA Civ 853). However, Mr Justice Hedley reminds us that there are 'very diverse standards of parenting and unequal consequences flowing from it … it is not the provenance of the state to spare children all the consequences of defective parenting' (Re L (Care: Threshold Criteria) [2007] 1 FLR 2050). There are a range of possibilities that flow from an assessment carried out under s.47. (See Working Together to Safeguard Children 2015.) If it has been difficult to gain access to Amelia to assess her, then the local authority may seek a Child Assessment Order (CAO, s.43), or if immediate action is necessary to protect her from danger, an Emergency Protection Order (EPO). Both of these orders involve applications to court. Strategy discussions between the multi-agency partners will enable a decision to be taken and advice from the local authority legal department will need to be sought. If the intervention made by the local authority in conjunction with the other professionals involved with the family does not ensure that Amelia is safeguarded from significant harm, then a decision to apply to court for a care order may be taken.

When an application is made to court by the local authority, they are required to follow the statutory guidance of court orders and pre-proceedings of local authorities (DFE 2014). This can be found at the website https://www.gov.uk/government/uploads/system/uploads/attachment_data/file/306282/Statutory_guidance_on_court_orders_and_pre-proceedings.pdf

The guidance outlines the duties placed on local authorities to identify concerns at an early stage and provide support to families. When it is decided that a child cannot continue to live with their parents, then there is a duty placed on the local authority to identify and prioritise suitable family and friends placements if this is appropriate. This is important because it may obviate the need to take care proceedings.

As record keeping and written evidence are very significant for court, social workers should always ensure that their recording of a case and the decisions made should be the best that they can be. Please see Chapter 2 on the importance of written communication skills. Cooper (2014) notes that in a case that goes to court the records of a case can be used to 'establish the "history" of the case and/or to judge the quality of the social work'. When a decision has been taken to apply to court because a child is suffering harm, it is important that the application to court should not fail because the quality of the social work involved is not evidenced in the records kept. Social workers need to be accountable for their decisions because of the impact they have on the lives of service users.

If a case does go to court because of the need to pursue a compulsory order, then social workers will be required to produce a written statement which as Cooper emphasises should be accurate and balanced because it will be scrutinised by the judge and the legal professionals representing both the local authority, the parents and the child. The following checklist should help social workers to focus on the skills needed to provide written evidence:

- Be clear what the statement is for and when it is needed by (timescales should be strictly adhered to otherwise a court order may be breached which is a serious matter).

- Provide a clear statement in your own words; you are the one who will be asked to justify it and may be challenged on it.

- Do not stray from the facts recorded in the case records. This is important because the records of a case also become court evidence and the statement should reflect this.

- Only give opinions that relate to your professional expertise and do not be tempted to stray beyond this.

- Follow advice from your legal department about how to set out your statement (Cooper, 2014).

When an application is made to court, the Public Law Outline (PLO, 2014) lays down the way in which judges should supervise the case from the beginning to end. It also promotes early engagement between parents and the local authority which is considering bringing proceedings and aims to encourage better applications and efficient court hearings. Annex 1 of the PLO lists the written evidence that is required to be provided when an application for a care or supervision order is made:

- Social Work Chronology.
- Social Work Statement and Genogram.

- The current assessments relating to the child and/or the family and friends of the child to which the Social Work Statement refers and on which the LA relies.

- Threshold Statement (summarising how the 'significant harm' threshold for making an order under s.31 Children Act 1989 is met).

- Care Plan.

- Allocation proposal form (the lawyers will specify which level of court the case should be heard in).

- Index of Checklist Documents: social workers are responsible for producing the first five documents.

Cooper (2014) highlights the importance of social workers being 'fully on top of the paperwork in the files and able to devote significant time to sorting the documentation and drafting a chronology, social work statement and geno-gram, threshold statement (social workers would normally draft this in close consultation with their legal adviser) and care plan'. The PLO gives guidance on what to include in the chronology, statement and genogram (Annex 1, 7.1).

Attending Court and Giving Evidence

Brammer (2015) notes that the key to a good experience in court is preparation, and gives a helpful summary of how to approach this preparation. Complying with the law and guidance above will go a long way to ensuring that social workers are well prepared for court, and this includes meeting with the local authority lawyers in advance of court attendance. In court, the judge is required to evaluate the evidence presented to him or her. To enable the judge to do so, the witness should be allowed to tell the court the story in their own words is (called examination in chief), and then allow the witness's evidence to be tested (called cross-examination) (Cooper, 2014).

The process of a social worker giving evidence is as follows:

1. The social worker enters the witness box and takes an oath or affirmation before giving his or her oral evidence.

2. The advocate representing the local authority's case conducts the examination in chief by asking the social worker to confirm the identity and contents of his or her statement.

3. The opposing advocate will then cross-examine the social worker with the aim of challenging and discrediting his or her evidence by proposing a different version of events.

4. Finally, the advocate that first called the witness has an opportunity to re-examine the social worker on any new points that have come up in cross-examination.

5. Then the judge or magistrate may ask some questions before the witness is able the leave the witness box.

Cross-examination is usually the dreaded part of giving evidence and is conducted by asking what are known as leading questions which are aimed at getting the answer that the advocate wants. As Cooper (2014) says 'it can be as long and short as a piece of string' and does not have to be limited to what was in the witness statement. The main advice at this stage is to attempt to stay calm and answer questions truthfully. Brammer (2015) advises on the importance of maintaining confident body language and addressing your answers to the bench (the judge and magistrates).

For further reading on the legal skills that social workers require when applying to court, see *Court and Legal Skills* by Cooper (2014).

Human Rights and Equality Considerations

Careful consideration of rights of service users provides a useful check on the excessive use of power on the part of social workers. The skill that social workers need to develop is to use their knowledge about the rights of service users to inform their professional judgement. In Amelia's situation, a rights-based approach can help with decisions about the risk to her whilst she remains within her family. Social workers should take into account the rights of all family members. The local authority has a duty to safeguard Amelia from harm and to ensure that there are no breaches of her Article 3 right not to be subjected to inhumane and degrading treatment. This may override her parents' Article 8 rights to a private and family life because any interference with their rights may be justified to ensure that she is safe from harm. It is important to remember that this is subject to the principle of proportionality. For example, if there was a decision about whether to apply for an EPO or a CAO, the local authority should be careful to take the decision which considered the rights of the whole family, and they should not go further in their actions than is necessary to achieve the outcome they wish to achieve for Amelia. In X Council v B (Emergency Protection orders) [2004] EWHC 2015 (Fam), the judge, giving guidance on the use of EPOs and CAOs, said that the court must 'scrupulously consider' the human rights of those involved and emphasised that the court's decision should be the decision that least interferes with the Convention rights of those involved.

Social workers would also need to be alert to the importance of ensuring that both Jane and Kamel were provided with support to be able to be meaningfully involved in the assessment and any subsequent decision. This requires sensitivity in the undertaking of the assessment and careful consideration of the need for an interpreter for Kamel and appropriate support for Jane. Failure to consider these issues would mean that the local authority could be deemed to have discriminated against Jane and Kamel and have not fulfilled their obligations under the equality duty. When undertaking an assessment which leads to a decision about Amelia and her parents' lives, Article 6, right to a fair trial, is engaged and it is important now and in any future court decision that the assessment is conducted fairly to ensure there are no breaches of the family's Convention rights.

Progress Check

The skills covered in this chapter should help you to understand how the legal framework empowers you to act in relation to service users and be aware of the duties that are placed upon you so that you can make judgements about what you have to do and what you may do (PCF 2.1 , PCF 5.2 and SoPS 13.4). Recognition of personal and organisational discrimination and the extent to which the law protects against this is vital to social work practice (PCF 3.2 and SoPS 2.6). Social workers need to be able to consider the rights of service users and ensure that any intervention that they make in their lives is lawful. There should be a recognition that this may result in a significant interference with the rights of some service users (PCF 4.2, 4.3 and SoPS 2.1).

Chapter Summary

Social work practice is highly regulated and there is a vast array of laws which apply to particular areas of practice. This chapter has focused on some key generic areas of law that apply to all social work practice and has offered guidance on how law can be applied in particular situations. What it is important to remember is that for each situation that calls for legal knowledge and skills, similar principles apply. Social workers need to have a working knowledge of the legislation, primary and secondary, cases and further guidance in order to make decisions that are legal and can be justified to service users, other partners and the courts.

Further Reading

- Brayne, H. , Carr, H. and Goosey, D. (2015) *Law for Social Workers*, 13th edition. Oxford: Oxford University Press.

  This book provides comprehensive and detailed coverage of the law that applies to social work practice.

- Cooper, P. (2014) *Court and Legal Skills: Palgrave Social Work Series*. Basingstoke: Palgrave Macmillan.

  Written by an academic and formerly practising barrister with years of experience in public law children's cases, this book provides social workers with the theoretical and practical knowledge they need to effectively deal with courts and legal issues, which includes presenting evidence, supporting vulnerable service users in the legal system and developing good professional relationships.

References

Brammer, A. (2015) *Social Work Law*, 4th edition. Harlow: Pearson Education
Brayne, H., Carr, H. and Goosey, D. (2015) *Law for Social Workers*, 13th edition. Oxford: Oxford University Press
Cooper, P. (2014) *Court and Legal Skills: Palgrave Social Work Series*. Basingstoke: Palgrave Macmillan.
Department for Education (2014a) Court Orders and Pre-proceedings for Local Authorities available at https://www.gov.uk/government/uploads/system/uploads/attachment_data/file/306282/Statutory_guidance_on_court_orders_and_pre-proceedings.pdf (accessed 21 June 2015).
Department for Education (2015a) Information Sharing: Advice for Practitioners Providing Safeguarding Services to Children, Young People Parents and Carers, available at https://www.gov.uk/government/uploads/system/uploads/attachment_data/file/419628/Information_sharing_advice_safeguarding_practitioners.pdf (accessed 21 June 2015).
Department for Education (2015b) Working Together to Safeguard Children, available at https://www.gov.uk/government/uploads/system/uploads/attachment_data/file/419595/Working_Together_to_Safeguard_Children.pdf (accessed 21 June 2015).
Health and Care Professions Council (2012) Standards of Proficiency – Social Workers in England, http://www.hpc-uk.org/assets/documents/10003B08Standardsofproficiency-SocialworkersinEngland.pdf (accessed 21 June 2015).
Johns, R. (2011) *Using the Law in Social Work*. 5th edition. London: Sage.
Ministry of Justice (2014) Public Law Outline, available at http://www.justice.gov.uk/courts/procedure-rules/family/practice_directions/pd_part_12a (accessed 21 June 2015).
TCSW (2012) Professional Capabilities Framework, http://www.tcsw.org.uk/pcf.aspx (accessed 21 June 2015).

Cases

Re A (A Child) [2012] UKSC 60.
Bull and another (Appellants) v Hall and another (Respondents) [2013] UKSC 73.
Re C (A Child) [2014] EWCA Civ 128.
HL v UK [2005] 40 EHRR 32.
Re L (Care: Threshold Criteria) [2007] 1 FLR 2050.

Re MA (Children) (Care Proceedings: Threshold Criteria) [2009] EWCA Civ 853.
P (by his litigation friend the Official Solicitor) (Appellant) v Cheshire West and Chester
    Council and another (Respondents) [2014] UKSC 19.
R v Islington Borough Council, ex parte Rixon [1997] ELR 66.
X Council v B (Emergency Protection orders) [2004] EWHC 2015 (Fam).
Re X (Emergency Protection Orders) [2006] EWHC 510.
YL v Birmingham City Council [2007] UKHL 27.
Z and others v UK (Application No 29392/95)(2001) 34 EHRR 97.

8

REFLECTIVE PRACTICE SKILLS

Carol Dicken and Dale van Graan

Introduction

This chapter aims to present a method to enable students to reflect on their practice, encouraging the integration and evaluation of knowledge (theory, research, legislation and policy) and practice through critical reflection. The chapter moves through the process of assessment, intervention and ending, enabling students to draw on case studies, their own life experiences and academic learning.

The chapter starts with a brief introduction to reflective practice before looking at the part that supervision can play in encouraging and developing students' and practitioners' critical reflective skills. Consideration is then given to the processes that learners and practitioners are likely to be following and then the place of their knowledge base in helping them to understand what they are doing and why they might be doing it. The section on discrimination, power and values assists students in using critical reflection to consider the impact of their own assumptions and the power dynamics at play within their practice. The chapter ends with a discussion of the way in which reflection can assist in identifying learning and development needs. Two case studies are provided in the chapter, which illustrate the levels of analysis and learning anticipated.

What is Reflective Practice?

There already exists a significant body of knowledge about reflective practice and its role in social work (Argyris and Schon, 1978; Boud et al., 1985; Schon, 1991; White et al., 2006; Thompson and Thompson, 2008; Knott and Scragg, 2013; Gardner, 2014) and so it will not be debated or redefined here. However, the approaches used, and which students and practice educators are encouraged to use, will be discussed through this chapter. For example, in our view, it is important to reflect for action, in action and on action (Thompson and Thompson, 2008).

Thompson and Thompson (2008) warn against adopting an oversimplified approach to reflective practice and usefully identify common misunderstandings arising from a range of theoretical perspectives. They describe reflective practice as a process of thinking or critically analysing which incorporates self-awareness, draws on knowledge and should lead to 'positive, emancipatory outcomes' (30). In developing the notion and role of self-awareness, it is suggested that reflective practice be viewed as a three-dimensional activity involving a complex interrelationship between the following components:

- *Cognitive*: thinking activities which are analytical, creative and 'deliberative' (33).

- *Affective:* exploring the emotional foundations and implications of our work, including sympathy and empathy, the role of emotional intelligence, dealing with anxiety and uncertainty, grief and the interrelationship between gender, culture and emotion.

- *Values:* specifically the notion of partnership, as it relates to work with service users and with colleagues in the same and in other disciplines, empowerment and equality and social justice.

Additionally, reflective practice needs to occur and take cognisance of the impact of the contexts in which it occurs, namely, the personal reflective, the supervisory and the group learning spaces (Thompson and Thompson, 2008). Each one of us has a personal, professional responsibility for critical reflection on our own practice and so the personal space could be seen to be the primary reflective context. This should then be developed through processes involving others as critical friends, such as in practice tutorials and supervision. Additionally, students and practitioners may also have opportunities to reflect and explore learning in groups, such as in student groups in placement, as team members in settings or in tutorial groups at university. There may also be other opportunities provided through attending training courses or specific learning events.

Practice Focus 8.1

During their placements all students are encouraged to develop the 'habit' of reflecting on practice, as well as their actual skills in critical reflection, by regularly recording their reflections and learning in a placement diary. Your practice educator may wish to have access to selected diary entries throughout the course of the placement. This should ideally be agreed in the Practice Learning and/or Supervision Agreement. You should have opportunities to create a personal space for reflection and to develop skills through discussion and specific formative feedback, whilst also providing the practice educator with a source of assessment of your reflective practice capability and evidence of your learning and development.

▶

◀ You may also draw on these diary entries when critically reflecting on the whole learning experience towards the end of the placement which, in turn, should also inform the review of your personal and professional development for the next placement or the Assessed and Supported Year in Employment.

It has been suggested that group reflective learning opportunities can promote 'double-loop learning' (Argyris and Schon, 1978). Consideration of multiple perspectives may increase flexibility and promote confidence in trying new ways of working. Double-loop learning may be deemed to have occurred when learners become self-directed, formulate principles drawn from their experiences and apply these to new situations. Assumptions may also change through this process. In contrast, single-loop learners are more likely to adjust their behaviour to accommodate the context. Double-loop learning may be an approach best suited to professions such as social work, with the challenge of highly complex work within constantly changing environments. It could be argued then, that practice educators have a responsibility to develop teaching approaches which will promote double-loop learning and that students and newly qualified social workers should aim to maximise their learning by adopting such an approach (TCSW, 2013).

Whilst this may be an appropriate goal for a final placement or students who bring an advanced level of critical reflection to their practice, one of the fundamental starting points for social work students is to learn how to use tools or models of critical reflection, such as Kolb's Experiential Learning Cycle (1975 in Knott and Scragg, 2013: 20). Kolb sees experiential learning as 'a process that links education, work and personal development' (Kolb, 1984: 4). This model proposes that effective learning is based on four kinds of ability which are applied in four stages of a learning cycle, namely concrete experience, observations and reflections, formation of abstract concepts and generalisations and testing implications of concepts in new situations. Kolb argues that 'learning is the process whereby knowledge is created through the transformation of experience' (Kolb, 1984: 38). This is only one of a number of models which can be used for reflective thinking and writing.

The introduction of the Professional Capabilities Framework (TCSW, 2012) has raised the profile of reflective practice, holistically embedding some reference in most domains across End of First Placement and Qualifying Social Worker level descriptors as well as Assessed and Supported Year in Employment (ASYE) and beyond. Additionally, there is specific reference to the role of supervision in relation to sustaining and developing reflective practice. In the level descriptors for End of First Placement (TCSW, 2012), supervision itself is mentioned specifically in Professionalism; however, the terms 'with guidance' or 'with support' are used in relation to values and ethics, diversity, rights, justice and economic well-being, knowledge, critical reflection and analysis, intervention and skills and contexts and organisations. It is reasonable to deduce that by virtue of their roles and the responsibilities associated with them, one of the people with responsibility for guiding and supporting a student's learning on placement is the practice educator or practice supervisor (TCSW, 2013). So how might supervision contribute to reflective practice?

The Role of Supervision in Reflective Practice

This section will identify the purposes of supervision in relation to practice education and to holistic assessment of learning and development (TCSW, 2012). The terms supervision and practice tutorial are used interchangeably, the former term generally denoting supervision provided by the practice supervisor or line manager, the latter specifically being the responsibility of the practice educator (or practice assessor for those undertaking post-qualifying training). Supporting a student to develop reflective skills may occur in both supervisory spaces. Shardlow and Doel (1996) suggest that supervision in a practice learning setting comprises four functions:

- education: guidance, teaching, evaluation of practice;

- pastoral: general awareness of support for the student's particular personal needs or difficulties;

- managerial: quality assurance of services to service users, maintenance of agency standards;

- administrative: organising and managing the placement.

Similarly, Hawkins and Shohet (2012) identify the three functions of professional supervision post-registration as *development, resourcing* and *qualitative*, whilst Wonnacott (2012) identifies *management, support, development* and *mediation*. Irrespective of the theoretical perspective adopted, it can be argued that supervision is one of the primary reflective spaces available to students and practitioners and through which assessment of learning and identification of support needs may be addressed. Where the development and education functions correspond, the focus is on enabling learners to develop skills, understanding and capacities through critical reflection on and exploration of interaction with service users and others. Critical questioning can promote increased self-awareness, critical examination of values and belief systems, critical analysis and evaluation of skills and knowledge applied and the exploration of new ways of doing, of thinking and of being.

The Practice Educator Professional Standards (TCSW, 2013) explicitly require practice educators, at both Stage 1 and Stage 2, to organise learning opportunities, enable learning and professional development and manage the assessment of learners within a clear and positive values framework. Enabling critical reflection is only one component of the teaching responsibility. It may be the one, however, which is most significantly affected by the nature of the teacher–learner relationship, in that it requires of the learner an openness to being 'exposed' or to risk demonstrating a lack of knowledge or skills, or values which do not fit with those of the profession. It may therefore lead to formative or summative assessment of insufficient capability. It is crucial for a safe, supportive, but sufficiently challenging learning environment to be created and sustained, within the supervisory relationship.

Maximising learning through the use of supervision could be seen to be the student or practitioner's responsibility. This may require specific preparation, an understanding of the goals and purposes of supervision and proactive use of critically reflective discussion. Follow-up activities such as reading, research or skills development may promote more embedded learning. It is likely that the practice educator will have a favoured supervision style, which will also need to take into account the student or practitioner's preferred learning style. What is key is the ability of the practice educator or supervisor to use a model to enable critical reflection such as Kolb's experiential cycle (1984) to raise a number of critical questions, which would enable the learner to progress through the cycle. This may not only promote learning through modelling, but also enable assessment of the learner's reflective skills. This is greatly facilitated by using a piece of reflective writing, either as a journal entry or a case analysis.

Case Study 8.1: **Martin's supervision**

Martin is a social work student on his first placement. He is 42 years old, married and has two school aged children. He is of Black African descent and has been living in England for the past ten years. His pre-course experience includes running a faith-based youth group and working as a support worker for people with mental health needs.

Martin has been placed at the Horizon Centre which provides day and outreach services to people with physical and learning disabilities. The centre has an active service user committee and aims to be service user led.

Martin has a practice supervisor, Karen, who is one of the assistant managers. She is a white English woman aged 34 and is also married with two young children. She has been working at the centre for the last five years and has supervised three students previously.

Martin also has an off-site practice educator who visits the placement fortnightly to support his learning and assess his development. Pamela is a Black British woman aged 45 who is a single parent of a teenage daughter. She has worked with Karen previously.

▶

After Martin had been in the placement for a number of weeks, Pamela noticed that he always appeared to be awaiting instructions. When told what to do by herself or Karen, he was very conscientious in carrying out tasks but seemed to lack initiative. She decided to raise this in supervision with him.

Pamela told Martin that she was pleased with the way that he was responding to the suggestions that she and Karen had made but she had observed that he did not appear to be bringing any of his own ideas for working with the service users. Martin initially felt hurt and criticised, although he was happy that Pamela recognised that he was doing what he had been told to do. He told Pamela that he did not feel sufficiently knowledge-able about the service user group to make suggestions. He also felt that as she and Karen were the teachers, they knew best.

Pamela helped Martin to reflect on what knowledge and skills he had gained from the university modules that could be applied to work with service users. They also discussed Martin's previous education experience and he identified that he had been taught to revere teachers and not to question what he had been told. This meant that he felt it was not his place to propose a course of action.

In thinking about this case study, ask yourself the following questions:

How could you use feedback from your practice educator to develop your practice?

What could your practice educator do to help you to be more reflective in supervision?

Case Study 8.2: **Georgina's supervision**

Georgina is a social work student on her final placement. She is 22 years old and is in a relationship with another woman. She does not have any children. She is a white woman of Irish descent. Her previous placement was in a Women's Refuge. Her pre-course experience was as a nursery assistant.

The placement is a statutory team working with children and their families.

Georgina has an on-site practice educator who is a trainee currently working towards Stage 2 of the Practice Educator Professional Standards. The practice educator, Meenah, is a British Asian woman aged 30 who is married and has a two-year-old child. She has been in the team since an organisational restructuring six months ago.

Georgina has been allocated several families to work with. She becomes aware that although she feels she is working well with the mothers and the children, she has not really engaged with the fathers. She decides to discuss this in supervision with Meenah.

Meenah asks Georgina to think about the skills she is using to engage with the mothers and children. She asks Georgina what is different about engaging with the fathers.

Georgina reflects on her visits and identifies that she always makes the arrangements with the women and that the men are rarely at home. If they have been there when she visits, they have gone into another room. She recognises that she has felt quite relieved about this as she is not very confident about working with men. Meenah and Georgina discuss her previous work and placement experience and how easy it could be for Georgina to view all men negatively.

Meenah and Georgina discuss some strategies to include the fathers in the assessments and intervention. Meenah also suggests that Georgina does some joint work with Tina who is another social worker in the team who is particularly good at engaging fathers. Georgina decides that she is going to use her reflective diary to think about how her own experience of family roles might influence her work with families.

How can you use supervision to identify areas of practice in which you are less confident?

How might your practice educator help you to develop critical thinking skills about all aspects of your practice?

Reflection on Social Work Processes

It is important to be continually reflecting on what we are doing as social workers, and one of the main areas for this is in working with people who use services as social workers assess, plan and intervene with them and their carers.

Different agencies and different groups of people who use services will require different procedures for assessment. There are also different stages at which assessment is required. Assessment is a continuous process and requires social workers to be aware at all times of the changes in the individual and their environment that may affect the person and their functioning. The process of reflection can help to identify those changes and whether they are likely to be of benefit or hindrance to the service user.

In reflecting on the assessment process, the task needs to be clearly identified. What is it that needs to be found out in order to assess the individual? There are some settings where it is necessary to gather a great deal of information; there are others where it is only the presenting issue and situation that are the focus. Knowing what the aim is at the start is a great aid to reflecting afterwards.

There may be a particular assessment form to complete for the agency, and it will be possible to consider, after information has been gained from the service user or others, how effectively assessment skills have been used. An assessment will usually involve working with the service user or carer to understand their perspective about the current situation. Consideration will need to be given to the use of a particular method of assessment, such as the procedural or exchange model (Smale et al., 2000), and how this affected the assessment process. It is important to think about the questions that were asked and how the person assessing responded to the information that was being shared. What was observed? Did the information that was given appear to be congruent with what is known about the service user or carer? People may wish to present themselves as managing better than they actually are and seeing how someone actually manages practical tasks may give useful information for an assessment. It is important to keep in consideration, however, that many people live with fluctuating psychological, social and medical conditions, and how they are functioning on the day of the visit may not be representative of their capability every day. It is therefore useful to reflect for action (Thompson and Thompson, 2008) in order to plan for meetings or contact with service users and carers and to anticipate potential challenges.

It is also necessary to reflect on the information that is received from others about the service user. Use critical thinking skills to identify where there are discrepancies in the views of different people and reflect on why this might be the case. How can the information gathered be assessed?

Practice Focus 8.2

Sometimes we are unaware of the extent to which we have been gaining information until we are reflecting on it. A student social worker had undertaken a home visit with the aim of working with the family's six-year-old daughter on an agreed direct piece of work. In supervision afterwards with her practice educator she shared how disappointed she was that she had not been able to complete this because of the number of family members present in the room. The practice educator, through reflective questioning, helped her identify what she had observed about the parents' interaction with the children during the visit. This gave relevant information about the quality of interaction and the student was able to recognise how much information she had gained during the visit.

Reflecting on what has been understood about the situation and the issues that need to change will help to identify which method of intervention is likely to be most helpful. Once the method has been chosen, and work has commenced, evaluation about how effective it is can be started. In order to do this, it is necessary to be clear about the aims of the intervention. It is difficult to reflect on whether progress is being made unless there is a plan. Either during a session with a service user, as *reflection-in-action,* or afterwards, *reflection-on-action* (Schon, 1991), reflection can help to consider the effectiveness of engagement skills and whether the person is fully engaged in the process. If not, what is it that is hindering this? Is the service user involved as a partner in the process? What is being done to give that message to the service user? If the social work approach that is being used requires working in partnership (as most do), how is this being done? It is also helpful to consider the intervention from the service user's perspective. How might they be feeling about working with the worker on the issues?

Practice Focus 8.3

When you have been using a particular method or approach consider the following:

How useful was the method in addressing the issues with this particular service user? What did it help you to do? Were there any disadvantages?

How proficient were you at using the method?

Finally, the ending process needs to be reflected on. How was the service user or carer prepared for the ending? Did it happen according to the plan or unexpectedly? What feelings did the ending engender and how might the service user be feeling about finishing either the session or the planned piece of work? If the intervention was starting again with the same service user, what was effective and what could be done differently?

Case Study 8.3: **Martin and the social work process**

Karen has asked Martin to talk to Brian, a 22-year-old white service user who has told her that another service user at the centre and living in the same group home has been calling him names. Martin talks to Brian and discovers that he is experiencing bullying and is not happy living in his current accommodation. Martin asks Karen to help him identify other more suitable accommodation for Brian. Karen is concerned that Martin has jumped to solution-finding without fully exploring the issues. She asks him to find out more about Brian's situation.

When Martin thinks about the exchange model of assessment, he realises that he has not fully explored Brian's experience and perspective. He heard the problem and Brian's wish to move and responded only to that. He realises that he has focused on the practical issue and did not ask Brian about how he is feeling. Martin actually feels a little out of his depth as he has never had to deal with an issue like this before. Karen has reminded him that he needs to work with Brian to fully understand his situation and share ideas about ways to move forward. After talking more with Martin, Brian says he does not really want to move, but that he does want the bullying to stop.

Pamela helps Martin to recognise that the ethos of the agency is compatible with a strengths-based approach and the exchange model of assessment. She asks Martin to find out more about the bullying and identify with Brian the risks and strengths of his current situation and different ways the problems could be addressed.

How can you reflect on your assessment of a person's needs and prioritise and plan intervention?

How might the practice educator help you to think about an assessment and possible intervention methods?

Case Study 8.4: **Georgina and the social work process**

Georgina has been working with Charlene aged seven and Andrew aged five and their parents to ensure that the children have a regular routine and are having their needs met. The children have recently come off a safeguarding plan following their mother Anne's successful community detox from heroin. Georgina has managed to get Peter (the children's father) to meet with her occasionally.

Although Anne appears to have engaged well with Georgina and seems to be receptive to her support, the school is still concerned about the children arriving late. Through her reflection Georgina has become aware that, although she has a positive relationship with Anne, this is not in itself sufficient to change Anne's parenting skills. She recognises that her intervention needs to be goal-oriented and purposeful and so puts this on the agenda for supervision. At university the lecturers had also talked about planning for endings and she knows that the team manager is keen to have this case closed as soon as possible.

Meenah asks Georgina what she thinks the purpose is of her intervention with this family and how far she has involved Anne and Peter in deciding what needs to be done or needs to change. She asks Georgina what method of intervention she is using and why. She asks her how she is taking account of new information in the process of a continuous assessment. Meenah reminds Georgina what the areas of concern were previously and what needs to be achieved in order to close the case. They discuss the possible conflict between the organisational thresholds for intervention and Georgina's desire to help Anne and Peter achieve the best for their children.

How might you reflect on the way in which you are undertaking an intervention with service users?

How might the practice educator enable you to build on this reflection?

Knowledge, Legislation and Policy

The HCPC Standards of Proficiency (HCPC, 2012a) and the Professional Capabilities Framework (TCSW, 2012) are both explicit about the need for social workers to be aware of their professional knowledge and be consciously using it in practice. This is relevant to reflective practice because it is necessary to think about how our knowledge base affects how we approach a case, engage with a service user, assess needs and plan for intervention. Thompson and Thompson (2008) borrow the term 'knowledgeable doer' from nurse education arguing that 'knowing and doing need to be connected' (22). Knowledge relevant to social work is likely to come from a range of different sources. There may be knowledge about the person who uses services and their family members on the agency files or within a referral. Other agencies may also have relevant information to share and reflecting on how this information contributes to the assessment is important. It is also possible, of course, that information gained from others is their opinion, rather than fact. It may also have been gained at a particular point in time when the situation of the person or family may have been different. Initial information gained prior to meeting a person who may need services is likely to start us to think about the person, what they may be like and what their needs may be. It may also raise issues that we need to be aware of regarding our own safety. Identifying our assumptions in a conscious manner means that we are able to check them out with the service user and they are less likely to lead to discrimination and prejudice.

It is likely that knowledge learned as part of a pre-registration social work programme will be relevant to understanding the context of social work practice. Collingwood (2008) suggests that theory can be divided into that which helps us to understand the person and their situation and that which helps us to decide how to intervene. It may be helpful, for example, to consider theories of human development and which ones might be relevant to the person. It is possible that events throughout a person's life may be having an impact on the current situation, so theories such as attachment (Bowlby, 1984) may be as relevant when working with older adults as when working with children. Howe (2008) argues that theory can be helpful in helping us to understand what we are seeing or what we are looking for, giving us a framework and the language to explain what we are seeing, helping us to consider what might be causing issues, predicting what might happen and the intervention that may be helpful.

Different social workers are likely to have their own views about why situations have occurred and this is likely to reflect whether they lean towards psychological or sociological theoretical explanations. Knowledge is not value-free and reflection on the theories that we prefer may help uncover personal assumptions. Thompson and Thompson (2008) make a distinction between *open knowledge,* which is exposed to the scrutiny of critical reflection, and *closed knowledge,* which is used without the same level of awareness and reflection. Eraut (1994) identifies the importance of *generalisation* in the development of both *conscious* and *semi-conscious* ways of working when one case appears to be similar to another. Organisations have some set procedures to be followed in certain situations and individual social workers will develop their own practices for intervening in particular circumstances, but Eraut recognises that professionals need to be aware of the danger of following *common practice* without engaging in a reflective process about whether there are matters that require a different way of working or issues that challenge individual or organisational values.

There has been an emphasis in recent years on 'evidence-based practice' and it is important for social workers to keep abreast of research relevant to their area of practice. This may give some evidence of what has been effective in other settings and new ideas of how to approach issues. It may also inform practitioners about what people who use services would find helpful. It is important to retain a critically reflective stance in considering the relevance of research evidence in helping social workers to work with people who use services in better and more productive ways.

Social workers also need to reflect on their knowledge of social policy and legislation and how this informs practice. What does a particular policy or piece of legislation indicate that the worker needs to do? New policies and new pieces of legislation may require that practice is changed. Research evidence may change policy and legislation. Situations will frequently occur throughout a social worker's career that necessitate updating knowledge of policy and legislation as this is ever-changing.

Practice Focus 8.4

How does my knowledge help me to understand the situation?

How does this knowledge influence what I plan to do?

What effect did it have on the outcome?

Not all sources of knowledge about how to do social work are from formal sources. As social workers practise they acquire knowledge about how to deal with situations and ways of working, and practice educators in particular will share this experiential knowledge with others. It still needs to be reflected on and evaluated, however.

Case Study 8.5: **Martin's knowledge**

In order to understand the bullying, Martin decides to read more about the Equality Act 2010 and how it might affect Brian. He also looks at the organisation's policies and discusses with Karen what his responsibilities are towards Brian and helping him keep safe. Karen suggests that he also looks at the policies of the agency that runs the group home and the National Care Standards.

Pamela asks Martin what he already knows about group living arrangements for adults with a learning disability and suggests he access the SCIE website and other resources to increase his knowledge. She also asks him about what he knows about personalisation and how this affects his approach to his work with Brian.

How might you reflect on what you need to know to work effectively with service users and carers?

What do you already know?

What else do you need to find out?

How can the practice educator support this process?

Case Study 8.6: **Georgina's knowledge**

Georgina identifies that she needs to know about drug use and recalled university teaching about the psychological and sociological factors of addiction. When prompted by Meenah she decides that she needs to read more specifically about the impact of drug use on parenting. She also recognises that, although she was using her knowledge about child development to help her assess the children's progress and needs, she needed to think more about how disruption to their routines might affect the children. This fits with the assessment framework used by the agency. Georgina is confident that she knows the relevant legislation and policy including the area safeguarding procedures and the agency eligibility criteria. Meenah asks Georgina to think about how this knowledge might help her to make a decision about the necessity for continued work with the family.

How might you develop a critical understanding of the application of knowledge in order to make decisions and work effectively with people?

How might practice educators enable this process?

Discrimination, Power and Values: Reflecting on Ethics and Values

Sometimes the first thing that becomes apparent when working in a new setting is the extent of the discrimination and oppression being experienced by people. Social workers may recognise their own attitudes and preconceptions and the way in which their views may have been formed by stereotypes. Reflecting on how these perceptions and attitudes can influence engagement with people, and assessments of their needs and circumstances, is vital for development of our practice.

People we are working with may be similar or different to ourselves in terms of gender, race, religion, ability, life experiences, class, sexuality, economic well-being or age. It is useful to reflect on how these differences affect not only how **we** approach and interact with people but also how **they** may view **us**. It is not always the case that differences make engagement more difficult and similarities make it easier. Assessing someone with a situation that is familiar to us because we have experienced the same issue may lead us to assume that they will feel the same as we did or react to it in a similar way. They may, however, follow a very different course than our own because of a range of factors. Using supervision to discuss these factors is an important part of critical reflection.

Practice Focus 8.5

A white male practice educator was working with a black female student. The cases allocated to her were predominantly white families because of the area in which the office was based. He allocated her an assessment of a black family from a similar background to her own. She completed the assessment and in supervision afterwards reflected that she had found this one of the most difficult families to assess. The practice educator was surprised and the student explained that she had felt pressure from the family to make allowances because of their shared culture. There was useful learning for both the student and the practice educator from this situation.

Social workers need to be aware of the power dynamics inherent in work with service users and carers. As gatekeepers of scarce resources, they may appear to others as having the power to distribute these at will. In reality, eligibility criteria and internal processes may appear to give little decision-making power. However, it will probably be the quality of assessments and communication of people's needs, whether by a report or face to face with a panel, that may determine resource allocation. When a funding application has not been approved, practitioners may feel powerless and can reflect on whether there was anything that could have been done differently. Was someone given too much expectation that a service could be provided? Has the service user's situation been relayed in sufficient detail?

In other areas of social work practice, power may be used to remove children from their birth families following safeguarding concerns or to place people in secure accommodation for their own safety or the safety of others. It is important to consider how we respond to these situations. The use of these powers is likely to have an emotional impact and social work students need to develop resilience without becoming hardened to people and their situations and being oppressive in practice. Reflection with honesty about the ethical dilemmas inherent in social work practice is one of the strategies for maintaining emotional intelligence and resilience. Kinman and Grant (2011) find that:

> Reflective ability appears to be an important predictor of resilience and psychological well-being, suggesting that trainee social workers who are better able to reflect on their thoughts, feelings and beliefs; who are able to consider the position of other people; and who can use these reflective abilities to communicate with others are more likely to be resilient to stress and be less distressed.
>
> (Kinman and Grant, 2011: 270)

Practice Focus 8.6

We need to develop an awareness of our own personal and professional values and how these influence the work we are doing.

Are your values in line with the professional value statements? What about the organisation's values? How do you reconcile any differences between your personal, professional and organisational value systems?

Why have you come into social work? Are you doing what you thought you would be doing to make a difference?

Dalrymple and Burke (2006) argue that 'the ability to be aware of one's values and to understand how they inform practice is essential in beginning to work anti-oppressively' (86). They go on to argue that critical practitioners need to be aware of their own values and the fact that they are participating in and not just observing the lives of others. It is essential to reflect on the way that values impact on the situations social workers are working with and the intended intervention. The issues that are important to the service user also need to be considered. How might they feel they are communicated with by social workers and by others? How much power do they have to change their situation? How much power do they feel they have to change the situation? Do they **feel** they have been treated or judged unfairly?

Case Study 8.7: **Martin and discrimination, power and values**

Martin initially assumed that the bullying Brian was experiencing was about his disability. In his further discussions with Brian, he starts to understand that the bullying is related to Brian's sexuality. From his reading about the Equality Act, he knows that discrimination about a person's sexual orientation and disability is illegal. He recognises that he feels more confident in addressing disablism than homophobia.

Pamela asks Martin to think about his personal beliefs and how these have been developed through his life experiences. Together they consider the social work values of ethical practice, valuing diversity and challenging discrimination.

Which of your attitudes and personal values might be challenged by your work with service users?

How prepared are you to discuss your personal and professional values with your practice educator?

Case Study 8.8: **Georgina and discrimination, power and values**

In a reflective commentary, Georgina considers how she has responded to working with Peter. She writes about her initial lack of confidence in engaging him and how this affected the work with the family. Following her discussions with Meenah in supervision, she recognises that this might be perceived as discrimination in terms of failing to include him in the process and in placing the full responsibility for parenting with Anne which might be perceived as sexist. Meenah has also helped Georgina to think about how she had perceived Peter as powerful but that he might see her as holding the power to make decisions about them and their children. Through this process, Georgina has become more aware of her power as a social worker and how she can use this constructively to promote partnership working.

What areas of potential or actual discrimination, power and values might you need to reflect upon? How confident do you feel about challenging discrimination and oppression? How might your practice educator help you to recognise potentially conflicting or competing values?

Identifying Continuing Learning and Development Needs

Whilst continuing professional development may be one of the functions of supervision (Wonnacott, 2012), the Professional Capabilities Framework is embedded in a clear expectation of individual ownership of and responsibility for identifying and pursuing continuing learning needs and contributing to the learning and development of others, throughout social work training and ongoing careers. With increased experience, the need for enablement of this process should diminish, but practice educators and supervisors are often best placed to facilitate the early development of these skills.

Placements usually commence with the expectation that a student has an understanding of their learning needs. It is important that these are articulated within your placement learning contract. However, it is this process of defining what it is that is unknown which can be particularly challenging, especially for those embarking upon a first placement. It is often at this point that students feel somewhat overwhelmed that they 'need to know everything about everything' to do with the placement. The practice educator can be helpful in enabling you to use the supervision space to 'tease out' your prior knowledge and experience, recognise your strengths and transferable skills and define the placement expectations. You can then be supported to identify your specific learning needs.

There is an expectation that practice educators and supervisors will provide students with clear, evidenced-based and balanced feedback about their strengths as well as areas for development (Shardlow and Doel, 1996; Williams and Rutter,

2013), in accordance with the requirements for each placement and the guidance on ethical practice (HCPC, 2012b). This should be a continuous process punctuated by specific assessment points, such as midway and end of placement.

Simultaneously, by using a range of reflective spaces, and taking account of a range of sources of feedback, students need to demonstrate capability in critically evaluating their practice (that is the doing, the knowing and the being) from different and multiple perspectives. By using a reflective model and being challenged by reflective questioning, students can demonstrate increased self-awareness and learning from multiple varied learning opportunities, identifying both their strengths and the areas in which they need or want to develop. Sometimes this can be a painful experience, as hearing others' perceptions, observations and experiences may challenge you to consider yourself in a new light. Others' feedback may differ from your self-view, positively or negatively. It may be difficult to think about how to develop skills or knowledge, challenge or change beliefs or, alternatively, develop a professional self-image. You may find it really difficult to accept positive feedback or recognise your strengths and so the challenge may be about you learning to recognise or even assert these.

Case Study 8.9: **Martin identifying learning and development needs**

Throughout his work with Brian, Martin has been identifying learning and development needs with the help of Karen and Pamela. He has learned to be more proactive in both his work with service users and in using supervision. Martin is beginning to feel more able to put into practice some of the skills and knowledge that he has been learning at university and through his reading. He has begun to reflect on his own value base and that of the profession and identify the potential for tensions.

In a three-way meeting with Karen and Pamela, Martin is encouraged to reflect on his continuing learning and development needs. He recognises that he needs to develop more confidence in challenging discrimination and in advocating for service users. He needs to continue to develop his own hypotheses about situations and use critical reflection and analysis to evaluate these.

In reviewing your progress over the course of the placement, can you identify your areas of learning and development so far? What do you still need to know, or know how to do, to be effective in your placement?

What have other people suggested that you need to develop further?

Completing a final placement successfully is likely to symbolise the end of a defined period of study. It may be difficult for you to look beyond that to the requirements of the Assessed and Supported Year in Employment (ASYE) and what this means for your continuing learning and development. It will be necessary to proactively include consideration of the demands of the first year in employment and the level descriptors (TCSW, 2012), when thinking about your continuing learning needs as you are about to join the workforce in a perhaps, as yet, unknown context. More lateral thinking may be required of the practice educator and the student when considering the transferability of skills and knowledge, personal strengths and learning needs and the ever-changing, uncertain and complex contexts in which social workers practice.

Case Study 8.10: **Georgina identifying learning and development needs**

Georgina reflects that she has developed her skills in working with children and their families. Joint working with Tina has helped her start to gain some confidence in working with men but she recognises that this is still an area she needs to continue to work on. Georgina wants to find a job as a newly qualified social worker in Children's Services and she and Meenah plan some shadowing of court work to give her some experience as this is something that Georgina has not yet had the opportunity to do. Meenah also helps Georgina to reflect that her future practice may include times when she needs to use her power and authority as a social worker and develop her emotional resilience.

How can you demonstrate your commitment to your own professional development? What is likely to be expected of you as a newly qualified social worker?

Have you thought about how you can continue to contribute to the learning and development of others?

Progress Check

It may be useful at this point to consider the following in relation to your own reflective practice:

- How confident do you currently feel in your ability to critically evaluate your practice and knowledge base?

- What knowledge informs your practice? How helpful is it and how might you identify what else you need to know?

- To what extent are you aware of the most helpful reflective model for *you* to use in practice?

▶

- How are you maintaining and developing your resilience? What helps you and what are the barriers?

- How can you use supervision and feedback from others in developing your practice?

- In your reflection do you regularly address issues around diversity, power, authority and ethics in your practice? How do you plan to deal with potential conflict with your own values?

Chapter Summary

- Reflective practice is a core critical component of learning to be a social worker and is embedded in the qualifying and continuing development framework.

- Constructive feedback from those who use services should be central to the process.

- Supervision should play an integral role in enabling critical reflection and facilitating learning, particularly in practice learning contexts.

- Critical reflection needs to encompass examination of the knowing, doing and being aspects of practice and should recognise both strengths and areas for development.

Further Reading

- Gardner, F. (2014) *Being Critically Reflective*. Basingstoke: Palgrave Macmillan.

- Knott, C. and Scragg, T. (2013) *Reflective Practice in Social Work*. Exeter: Learning Matters/Sage.

- Thompson, S. and Thompson, N. (2008) *The Critically Reflective Practitioner*. Basingstoke: Palgrave Macmillan.

References

Argyris, C. and Schon, D. (1978) *Organisational Learning: A Theory of Action, Perspective.* Reading, MA: Addison-Wesley.

Boud, D, Keogh, R. and Walker, D. (eds) (1985) *Reflection: Turning Experience into Learning.* London: Routledge Falmer.

Bowlby, J. (1984) *Attachment and Loss. Attachment,* Vol 1. London: Penguin Books.

Collingwood, P. (2008) The Theory Circle: A Tool for Learning and for Practice. *Social Work Education,* 27 (1): 70–83.

Dalrymple, J. and Burke, B. (2006) *Anti-oppressive Practice: Social Care and the Law.* Maidenhead: Open University Press.

Eraut, M. (1994) *Developing Professional Knowledge and Competence.* London: Falmer Press.

Gardner, F. (2014) *Being Critically Reflective* Basingstoke: Palgrave Macmillan

Hawkins, P. and Shohet, R. (2012) *Supervision in the Helping Professions,* 4th edition. Maidenhead: Open University Press.

Health and Care Professions Council (2012a) *Guidance on Conduct and Ethics for Students.* London: HCPC.

Health and Care Professions Council (2012b) *Standards of Proficiency.* London: HCPC

Howe, D. (2008) Relating Theory to Practice. In Davies, M. (ed.), *The Blackwell Companion to Social Work,* 3rd edition. Oxford: Blackwell Publishing.

Kinman, G. and Grant, L. (2011) Exploring Stress Resilience in Trainee Social Workers: The Role of Emotional and Social Competencies, *British Journal of Social Work,* 41: 261–275.

Knott, C. and Scragg, T. (2013) *Reflective Practice in Social Work* 3rd edition, Exeter: Learning Matters/Sage.

Kolb, D. (1984) *Experiential Learning.* New Jersey: Prentice Hall.

Schon, D. (1991) *The Reflective Practitioner: How Professionals Think in Action,* 2nd edition. Aldershot: Arena.

Shardlow, S. and Doel, M. (1996) *Practice Learning and Teaching.* Basingstoke: Macmillan Press.

Smale, G., Tuson, G. and Statham, D. (2000) *Social Work and Social Problems: Working Towards Social Inclusion and Social Change.* Basingstoke: Palgrave Macmillan.

The College of Social Work (2012) *The Professional Capabilities Framework.* London: TCSW. Online, available at tcsw.org.uk/pcf.aspx.

The College of Social Work (2013) *The Practice Educator Professional Standards.* London: TCSW. Online, available at https://www.tcsw.org.uk/uploadedFiles/TheCollege/Social_Work_Education/PEP%20standardsand%20guidance%20update%20proofed%20and%20final%20021213.pdf.

Thompson, S. and Thompson, N. (2008) *The Critically Reflective Practitioner.* Basingstoke: Palgrave Macmillan.

White, S, Fook, J. and Gardner, F. (eds) (2006) *Critical Reflection in Health and Social Care.* Maidenhead: Open University Press/McGraw-Hill Education.

Williams, S. and Rutter, L. (2013) *The Practice Educator's Handbook* 2nd edition. Exeter: Learning Matters/Sage.

Wonnacott, J. (2012) *Mastering Social Work Supervision.* London: Jessica Kingsley Publishers.

9

SKILLS FOR LEADERSHIP

Keith Davies and Jeremy Ross

Introduction: Why Leadership?

Leadership has been the subject of intense concern, reflection and learning in social work in recent years. For example, rightly or wrongly, social work leaders have been the subject of particular criticism following serious case reviews (Laming, 2009; Jones, 2014). The Social Work Task Force (2009) devoted a chapter in its final report to the leadership of the profession and recommended the creation of the recently disbanded College of Social Work (2012) with such leadership in mind. Munro (2011) in her review of child protection argued the need for social work managers and practitioners to be led less by compliance with bureaucratised systems and more by professional judgement (5). However, notwithstanding this current preoccupation with leadership, a question might still arise regarding the relevance of a chapter on this subject in a book about skills for social work practice when leadership is most often identified as primarily a management concern. Two important sources help in addressing this question. Firstly, turning to Munro (2011) again, she argues that:

> leadership is often only understood in terms of individuals at the top of the hierarchy, but it is much more than the simple authority of one or two key figureheads. Leadership behaviours should be valued and encouraged at all levels of organisations. At the front line, personal qualities of leadership are needed to work with children and families when practising in a more professional, less rule-bound, way.
>
> (107)

Challenging the profession to think about leadership differently, Munro identifies leadership qualities and behaviours as playing a key role at the heart of direct work with service users. At the same time and in line with this understanding of leadership, the Professional Capabilities Framework (PCF) includes professional leadership as one of its nine core domains. Social workers throughout their careers from entry into training onwards will develop their skills in each of the PCF domains, and the clear implication of the inclusion of leadership is that it is relevant and vital to all social work roles and to each stage in career development. As Hafford-Letchfield (2009) confirms:

> Leadership is a term that we tend to equate with positions of power, influence and status. However, acts of leadership can be observed at all levels of the organisational structure.
>
> (22)

Since leadership is widely 'distributed' across roles in this way (Lawler, 2007: 134), it is important to think about what leadership is in social work practice, to identify the sorts of skills involved in leading well and to formulate a plan for personal development in this domain.

Reflective Exercise 9.1

Thinking about your practice experience so far, identify those colleagues whom you have experienced as effective leaders. What roles did they occupy and what was it about their personal qualities and their behaviour which meant that you thought of them as leaders?

Turning to your own personal practice, which of the things you do might be described as leading? (For example, making decisions or leading by example.) Think about those occasions on which you influence other people in some way.

What is Leadership?

Although at face value leadership can seem a fairly simple idea and one which is understood in similar ways by most people, it is, on closer examination, elusive and contested (Lawler, 2007). As indicated above (Munro, 2011), the 'common sense' understanding of leadership tends to associate it with prominent, often heroic, individuals, usually men, whose innate charisma, authority and force of personality allow them to drive great changes and to motivate large groups of people. This 'Great Man' theory of leadership is related to psychological 'trait theory' in locating within the individual a set of inborn and consistent characteristics compatible with leadership (Lawler and Bilson, 2010; Northouse, 2013). As a template for leadership, this concept can be susceptible to romanticisation (Lawler, 2007: 125) and, it is suggested, is also somewhat removed from the image of themselves held by the majority of social workers.

Related to this 'Great Man' approach is a common association between leadership and the senior roles within an organisation. Although leadership is undoubtedly required in these roles, the identification of leadership solely with senior managers runs the risk of draining other social work roles of their proper leadership elements. In addition, it exacerbates a tendency to conflate the concepts of leadership and management whilst in fact there is still much debate regarding the extent to which they refer to separate things (McKitterick, 2015: 3). Indeed, the task of detailing more generally what leadership is has proved so challenging that Lawler and Bilson (2010) have argued that 'no comprehensive definition' (35) of leadership is likely to emerge.

Whilst recognising the general difficulty with the term 'leadership', this chapter adopts Northouse's (2013) understanding of it as:

> a process whereby an individual influences a group of individuals to achieve a common goal.
>
> (5)

This formulation envisages leadership not so much as a set of personal characteristics or traits but rather as an interaction between individuals. As Northouse (2013) further explains, the focus on leadership as a 'process':

> implies that a leader affects and is affected by followers. It emphasizes that leadership is not a linear, one-way event, but rather an interactive event. When leadership is defined in this manner, it becomes available to everyone.
>
> (5)

Despite the conceptual difficulties referred to above, some progress has also been made in untangling leadership from management. For example, Lawler and Bilson (2010) begin to distinguish management from leadership by associating the former with complexity and the latter with change. That is, despite an overlap between the two activities, management draws more on those organisational skills needed to coordinate activity, solve difficult problems and deliver services, whilst leadership utilises the ability to understand the wider environment to identify a direction, foster a culture, motivate people and illicit their commitment. In line with this framework, Hafford-Letchfield (2009) talks of the capacity of leadership to create:

> a belief in common purpose and to achieve a quality of life in the organisation that will generate and sustain commitment.
>
> (26)

Pertinently for social work she goes on to suggest that in stable times, management might be largely what is needed, but that in times of change, challenge and turbulence, it is leadership which is especially required. With change characterising social work organisations far more than stability in recent times, the need for leadership is all too apparent. Applying this idea to work with service users where situations are so often changeable and challenging as well as complex, it seems clear that practitioners too will need to use leadership as well as management skills.

Leadership Theory

In thinking about leadership skills for social work practice, the 'Great Man' and 'distributed' theories of leadership, touched on very briefly above, help to sharpen our sense of what leadership is and, hence, to clarify which skills might be needed when exercising it. Attention will now be turned to a range of other theoretical developments, ideas and models with a view to identifying those which are most relevant for social work and which shed most light on leadership skills in practice. Whilst the scope of the chapter prevents either a comprehensive or an in-depth study of leadership theory, nevertheless some important ideas will be discussed and indications for further reading given which the interested reader might follow up.

A corollary of the view that leadership skills are largely innate in exceptional individuals is that there is little scope for learning them. A social worker might discover latent leadership ability and this might be especially likely to occur if they have previously thought of leadership as a matter for other people who are essentially different from themselves. However, there will be scant grounds for systematically teaching and learning leadership.

By contrast, Binney et al. (2012), explicitly rejecting a 'Great Man' mindset, talk instead of 'living leadership' (xi). This is something much more ordinary, more widely exercised and, interestingly, far closer to direct social work practice itself. As Binney (2012) notes,

> it is what happens between people in a particular moment or situation. Leadership is a social process – the result of interactions between and within individuals and groups.
>
> (4)

The focus here is on what Lawler (2007: 126) describes as the 'nearby leaders' with whom social workers might share offices and encounter in everyday practice. Rather than a heroic activity undertaken by the exceptional, Binney et al. (2012) offer a vision of leadership as something carried out by 'ordinary' people, embedded in familiar social situations as they relate to each other. They also see it very much as a skill which can be learned, a view shared by Northouse (2013).

Taking these ideas of leadership through relationship a little further, Lawler (2007) refers to what has become known as 'transactional leadership'. Here, the relationship between leader and follower is seen in terms of transactions between individuals governed by incentives and self-interest whereby each is 'doing something in return for some form of reward' (127). The sort of leadership evoked here mirrors aspects of scientific management in which leaders arrange incentives and disincentives to achieve compliance and effort amongst followers who are regarded as resistant (Morgan, 1997: 22). It is pertinent here to think of those situations in social work practice in which certain valued behaviours on the part of service users might be encouraged or led not only through incentives but also through frank discussions about the consequences of failure to produce them. Lawler (2007) goes on to contrast this transactional approach to leadership with what has been termed 'transformational' leadership characterised by,

> encouraging major change through charisma, inspiration, individual attention and stimulation.
>
> (127)

The leadership described here is, like transactional leadership, directed towards changes in behaviour, but these are arrived at more through the vehicles of partnership, relationship and the embodiment of values. In the context of working with colleagues, Lawler and Bilson (2010) describe transformational leadership in terms of their ability to inspire, to motivate, to take a personal interest and, in so doing, to encourage others to take responsibility and to engage in positive activity.

These ideas of leading through attentiveness to individual concerns and through supporting motivation are not only a far cry from the popular conceptions of leadership described above but also much more akin to the personal practice most social workers would recognise and own. The same might be said of the 'servant and partnership' model of leadership developed by Alimo-Metcalf and Alban-Metcalf (2005) and which, as Cullen (2013) notes, places a particular emphasis in leadership on the ability to nurture and stimulate the development of others. In a more detailed account of 'Servant Leadership', Northouse (2013) describes how 'servant leaders':

> place the good of followers over their own self-interests and emphasize follower development ... They demonstrate strong moral behaviour toward followers ... the organization and stakeholders.
>
> (220)

There is a clear congruence between this way of leading and social work values such as respect, autonomy and empowerment.

It is clear then that leadership can be thought of in ways which are inclusive of front-line social workers and which reflect, surprisingly closely, what might be thought of as good social work practice. However, even when constructed as transformational, leadership is defined by influence over other people and is thus inextricably bound up with power (Northouse, 2013: 5). Taking this further, Northouse distinguishes between two forms of power: 'position power' and 'personal power'. The former derives from a formal role, the authority it carries to act and the discretion to allocate rewards, whilst the latter stems from knowledge, personal legitimacy and relational warmth (2013: 10). Social workers have position power deriving from the role, duties and powers ascribed to them by law but, at the same time, can generate personal power in their relationships with service users through their reliability, their knowledge and the care they demonstrate. It follows that, holding these powers of influence, social workers must be vigilant to avoid abusing them. In this connection, Northouse (2013: 11) is careful to separate leadership which he associates with influence 'towards a common goal' from coercion where others are induced to act against their own wishes and inclinations. Even when using power to influence a family and to lead towards increased well-being, social workers must be vigilant to do so in ways which are congruent with ethical principles. Even more so when using powers strongly and against the will, for example, of parents to achieve safety for their children, they will be heavily reliant on values to avoid abusive leadership.

Case Study 9.1

Martine is a social worker in a Community Mental Health team and has been qualified for three years. She works with health professionals such as community psychiatric nurses and psychologists as well as psychiatrists and other social workers. She is working with Brian, who is enrolled on a recovery programme run jointly by the local Community Care NHS Trust and an Adult College following a period of relapse in his bipolar disorder. The recovery programme consists of sessions or classes as well as individual support laid on at Adult Education Centres rather than at premises labelled as providing services for people with mental health issues.

Brian lives in a housing association flat and does not want his mother involved in his care as he finds her oppressive, stopping him living the life he wants. He is reluctant to take medication prescribed for him as he finds that it makes him feel flat and lifeless.

Martine has developed a positive relationship with Brian. She is aware that he enjoys writing poems and having his friend Shamir sing them to his sitar. She is encouraging Brian to describe his experiences, enrolling on a creative writing and songwriting class at the Recovery Centre.

At their last meeting, Martine told Brian that she wanted the Team she was working in to learn more about what Recovery meant. How, she asked, could Recovery 'be made real' to them? Brian read out a poem about his experience and how the Recovery Centre gave him a platform from which to rebuild his life. She asked him if he would be willing to allow her to read it at a team meeting. Brain asked if he could bring Shamir to sing the poem.

1 How is Martine showing leadership in her work with Brian?

2 Identify which of the concepts of leadership discussed above most closely reflect her practice in this case?

3 How is she using her power to influence others?

4 Are there further ways in which Martine might exercise leadership in her work with Brian?

In this brief consideration of leadership theory, the focus turns to the relationship between leading and identity. Here, even a moment's reflection reveals that culturally prevalent images and perceptions of leadership are loaded with gendered, racialised and other diversity-related meaning. For example, it will not have escaped the reader's notice that the term given to the model of leadership which emphasises inborn qualities of charisma, drive and force of personality is known as the 'Great Man' model. This model of leadership remains prevalent in many fields of employment and it has been argued that, in the public services, the sorts of leadership fostered by managerialist organisational cultures can tend towards the aggressive, competitive and driven (Thompson, 2011). Indeed, the persistence of a fairly robust 'glass ceiling' resisting women's entry into the highest leadership roles suggests a deeper, ongoing cultural difficulty in reconciling women and leadership. As Lawler (2007: 126) points out, gender-aware models of leadership have begun to develop only recently. With this in mind, social workers might find that distributed, living and transformational models of leaders sometimes need to find ways of flourishing within 'Great Man' organisational and wider cultures.

Since social workers practise in a range of organisations and settings, it is necessary here to acknowledge more explicitly the impact which those organisations have on leadership behaviour. As Binney et al. (2012) and Lawler (2007) point out, organisations and their ways of operating shape the ways in which leadership is expressed within them.

> The social and political, the business situation and the culture of an organisation (its characteristic patterns of thinking and behaving) shape the type of leadership that is given.
>
> (Lawler, 2007: 125)

Social work organisations are responsible for the culture of leadership which social workers experience, just as, for example, Anita Roddick is for the Body Shop:

> I run my company according to feminine principles – principles of caring, making intuitive decisions and not getting too hung up on hierarchy ... having a sense of work as being part of your life, not separate from it; putting your labour where your love is.
>
> (In Morgan, 1997: 136)

Organisations in which social workers practise also exist within political, legal and business discourses which interact robustly with professional ones. Therefore, despite the scope which social workers enjoy to define and develop their ways of leading, the space they have to do so is partly governed by the style of leadership encouraged or even required by the agency which employs them. In other words, leadership is to an important extent 'situational' (Binney, 2012: 7).

Finally, whilst considering leadership, diversity and situated practice, it is pertinent to reflect on the response of the social work profession to different leaders. For example, studies in ethics and diversity trace the historical location of leadership in Western cultures not only predominantly with men but also with white, able-bodied, middle and upper class, heterosexual men (Delgardo and Stefancic, 2012). As a result, despite sustained professional attention to anti-oppressive practices, it remains a challenge for social work to recognise and respect leadership across the range of identities, not least the leadership of service users and carers (see Chapter 4). In a slightly different way, it will also be important to keep in mind the various ways in which different cultural traditions construct leadership (Hofstede, 2003; Gast and Patmore, 2012). Both service users and colleagues drawing on different cultural heritages might carry contrasting expectations about the relationship between leaders and followers.

Case Study 9.2

You lead a team of social workers involved in the discharge from hospital of older people often recovering from strokes. An immediate task is to lead a discussion within the social work team of a new policy proposed by the clinical stroke team promoting prompt discharge at the point when recovery no longer requires a hospital environment followed by home-based rehabilitation. You are aware that clinicians and managers feel under pressure to free beds at an early date to help them to meet performance targets.

The relationship between the hospital social work team and both clinical colleagues and the hospital management has been strained at times. Recently, the local paper highlighted delayed discharges from the hospital and senior clinicians appeared to blame social workers for failing to arrange appropriate social care in a timely way. There has been a previous incidence of hostility between a clinical stroke lead and a social worker relating to a disagreement over the management of a patient's care. This has not been acknowledged or dealt with.

You recognise that members of the all-female social work team feel caught between the requirements of clinical and managerial staff on the one hand and, on the other, the shortage of resources in the community. They are reluctant on ethical grounds to agree discharge plans before services are in place. One team member has personal experience of severe difficulties arising following the discharge of a parent from hospital and has yet to come to terms with her feelings about this.

1 What type of leadership are you called upon to exercise in this meeting?

2 How might you exercise leadership regarding the team member with negative, personal experiences of discharge practice and the team member who was previously in conflict with the Clinical Stroke Lead?

3 How might you best lead in an anti-oppressive way?

Developing Leadership Skills in Social Work

Understanding leadership less as a combination of inborn characteristics and more as a set of behaviours used in the course of everyday situations and transactions between people locates it very much within the sphere of skills which can be learned and developed. In this section, attention turns to those skills, the exercise of which make up leadership behaviour, and an opportunity is provided for the reader to think about those which they already deploy well and others with which they would like to make further progress. At risk of defining leadership too broadly and hollowing out its meaning, we will think of developing leadership skills firstly in terms of the self, secondly in relation to work with service users and finally in the context of colleagues and team membership. This section will conclude by considering the light shed on the development of leadership skills by Katz's (1955) classic identification of technical, human and conceptual skill types.

Leadership of oneself is arguably a crucial part of the continuum which makes up leadership overall and represents a helpful place to start in developing leadership skills (McKitterick, 2015). Self-knowledge and awareness of personal strengths, vulnerabilities, identity and learning needs are perhaps best developed through proactive use of reflection and supervision. In terms of leadership, such self-awareness can lead to positive choices regarding learning experiences and an informed sharing of roles within a team to maximise strengths and contributions. It can also support knowledge of personal emotional triggers and form a foundation for the sort of emotional self-regulation under pressure in practice which marks out safe and effective leadership.

Self-leadership, as Mantell (2013: 87) argues, also requires a willingness to be visible, the courage to take responsibility for exercising power (even in the form of expressing a view, making a decision or suggesting a way forward) and the resilience to face criticism when others disagree or when things do not go according to plan. Self-leadership might be thought of as accepting this burden of responsibility for the good of the team and of service users.

Taking personal responsibility for dependability, good time-management, punctuality and prioritisation, some of the familiar professional skills, is also associated with self-leadership. Certainly those exercising this responsibility create a model for colleagues and service users and lead in this way. Developing leadership skills here might involve identifying personal learning needs, making a plan, seeking relevant training and using supervision.

Finally with regard to leading oneself, the deepening of knowledge can result naturally in leadership as practitioners turn to a colleague who has made the effort to become expert in an area. As practice throws up the need to learn more about procedures, a condition, the law or an aspect of theory, motivated social workers can undertake the research which allows them to be confident in that regard and to legitimately take the lead in hypothesising and problem-solving.

Turning to work with service users and carers, again there is a wealth of opportunity to develop leadership skills. For example, punctuality, respect, effort, the communication of hope and keeping one's word contribute powerfully to leadership in relationship with service users. It is a commonplace but nevertheless supported by evidence (Miller and Rollnick, 2002) that attitudes and actions communicate very directly and powerfully and the example of practitioners in their behaviour will offer a strong lead and model to service users and carers (Trotter, 1999).

Practitioners can also lead by making use of their knowledge to offer an assessment of a practice situation and a plan to solve or ameliorate problems and distresses. Again, by proactively using training and supervision and by consistently reflecting on their practice, social workers can foster their skills in using knowledge to offer a lead to service users. At the same time, a practitioner confident in their ability to lead might also be more able to share leadership with service users and carers and to be willing to co-lead with them wherever possible. However, it should also be acknowledged that leading work with service users can, where risk of serious harm is present or potentially so, involve asking the difficult questions, being transparent regarding intentions and possible outcomes and setting boundaries in highly charged circumstances. The skills of assertiveness, persistence and resilience called for might best be achieved in supervised practice with successively more challenging work. Careful reflection, observation of good models and supportive supervision are needed to nurture skills.

Finally, it will immediately be apparent that team membership also offers opportunities for the development of leadership skills. Chairing and minuting meetings, offering training, taking responsibility for particular initiatives or administrative tasks and acting up in the team leader's absence are just some examples. Thinking a little more broadly, acting as lead practitioner in a team around a child or family also requires significant leadership skill. In both settings, social workers may need to lead by challenging discrimination and thus shaping the working culture and, sometimes, by taking responsibility for saying the difficult thing to prevent group collusion with the line of least resistance. There will be a need as lead worker to create a vision for the work and to engage in motivation and advocacy in order to sustain that vision. Social workers developing their capacity to lead might seek out and observe good models and mentors whilst, at the same time, gradually taking on successively more prominent leadership roles themselves.

In order to anchor these suggested opportunities and methods for the development of leadership skills in social work a little more firmly, attention now turns to academic work regarding skills for leadership. Northouse (2013), in a summary of the literature addressing skills-based approaches to leadership, refers to Katz's (1955) early division of leadership skills into three broad categories, technical, human and conceptual (46).

Technical leadership skills concern competence in carrying out the tasks relating to specific roles and settings. For example, a clear grasp of relevant law, agency policy, resources, other agencies and IT will enable a social worker to proceed confidently and purposefully with a piece of practice and, in so doing, to offer a lead. Lacking confidence, for example, in assessment or referral process or being hazy about guidelines can impair leadership through hesitancy and delay. Depending on temperament, the learning of technical skills can present as hard work and even daunting. However, given a diligent effort, it rewards the social work practitioner by allowing them to accomplish core tasks quickly and accurately whilst supporting them in leading meetings with service users and other professionals through the clear contribution of accurate, relevant information. Taking the initiative to seek knowledge from documentation and from experienced colleagues is a clear step towards the development of technical leadership skills and helps others to have confidence in you as a leader.

Human leadership skills are, perhaps, those most readily recognisable by social workers as part of their core repertoire. Concerned with working with people, they include good communication and the fostering of trust, commitment and motivation. At the same time, they involve the management of the self and the sustaining of a joint endeavour through obstacles, conflict and the various forms of adversity. As they use these skills, social workers lead by engaging service users (and colleagues) personally in a plan of work and by carrying through that plan, despite discouragement and distraction, to the best conclusion available. Important leadership behaviours are involved here in initiating action, generating energy, holding course whilst others might be inclined to give up and jointly solving problems as they arise. With regard to learning communication and engagement skills for leadership, the reader is referred to Chapter 1 and, in particular, to the taking of opportunities to learn from the modelling of others and from feedback on personal performance. Also relevant is Chapter 8 and learning to use reflection and supervision to cope with fluctuations in motivation (one's own and that of others) and to develop resilience in seeing work through despite difficulties.

Closely related to these human leadership skills of communication and motivation are those of nurturing growth in others and developing emotional intelligence. Most clearly in formal supervision, but also in informal contact with colleagues and in work with service users, social workers are often involved in leading by supporting personal growth in others. At the most basic level, this might be through acting as an example and a role model. More consciously, it might be through informal case discussion or the offering of training inputs into team meetings. The skill concerns the communication of belief in others as well as the offering of information. The humility to take a back seat and delegate appropriately whilst others begin to develop and practice new skills are related leadership skills.

Perhaps another way of describing human leadership skills is to think of them in terms of emotional intelligence (Hafford-Letchfield, 2009; Lawler and Bilson, 2010). Emotional intelligence is characterised by Goleman (1998) as being made up of five core elements: 'Self awareness, Self Regulation, Empathy, Motivation, Social Skills'. In leading, social workers are consistently aware of and simultaneously managing their own emotional responses and those of others to maintain relationship through challenges and to steer practice. In learning emotional intelligence, once again, the modelling of others and the honest, purposeful use of supervision are valuable resources.

Finally, conceptual leadership skills are those involved in working with ideas (Northouse, 2013: 46). Leaders, whether in formal leadership roles or not, tend to have a clear vision of what the organisation, the team or an individual or family is fundamentally trying to achieve and their clarity of mind lends a framework to others for directing their practice. Values are one pivotal source of vision and social workers can lead in a wide range of situations by bringing the values dimension to the fore and by using it to shed light on problems and to create direction (see Chapter 3). Theory, combined with critical thinking and analytical skills, can similarly generate leadership in meetings, interviews, conferences and reports by offering a coherent, transparent framework in which those involved might conceptualise the situation and ways forward. (The reader is referred to Chapter 5 and the development of assessment skills.)

Case Study 9.3

Jenny is a social worker in an Initial Referral Team in Westchester Children and Community Services Department. This team consists of a Team Manager, two Senior Practitioners and five Social Workers. She has been in post for nine months.

As part of her Assessed and Supported Year in Employment, she has been developing ways in which the team might improve its approach to young women in abusive relationships. This has included setting up a Steering Group of young women referred to the team as well as representatives of other stakeholders. This project has been agreed between Jenny and the Team Manager following an increase in referrals of young women living in abusive relationships.

Jenny developed an interest in working with young women experiencing domestic violence during her final practice placement in a counselling agency for self-harming young people. She noticed a pattern of increased referrals from the Domestic Violence Unit at Westchester Police Station and social workers in Westchester Hospital Accident and Emergency Department as well as from young people themselves. She discussed this pattern with her manager in supervision.

Jenny has agreed to update her colleagues on progress in forming the Steering Group and beginning to advise on best practice. Not all team members are as yet convinced that young women in these circumstances are a priority service user group. Jenny is concerned that, as the newest and youngest member of the team, colleagues will not be completely supportive of her making suggestions for practice.

1 Making use of the models of leadership outlined earlier in this chapter, consider the types of leadership which Jenny has shown in relation to this practice initiative for young women described above. How has the Team Manager demonstrated leadership?

▶

2 Is there a potential in the team meeting for discriminatory practice to occur? If so, in what ways might it occur and how might it be avoided?

3 Which leadership skills will Jenny need to demonstrate most as she seeks to establish and to develop this service?

In summary, the following tables are designed to give some indications of how leadership skills might be developed (Table 9.1 and 9.2):

Table 9.1 Some opportunities for professional leadership at pre-registration level

In training and education	In practice	As citizen
Student representative on liaison/review committees, academic or programme boards	Chairing team meetings	Active membership of political party/engagement with political challenge
Mentoring other students	Presenting issue, theory/research or case to team	Active membership of community-based action group
Ambassadors for the institution	Representing team at multi-disciplinary meeting	Active support to others
Take responsibility for identifying own learning needs and planning to meet them	Taking responsibility for identifying own learning needs and planning to meet them	Maintain HCPC standards of ethics in personal conduct and taking opportunities to develop knowledge and skills

Table 9.2 Some opportunities for professional leadership at post-registration level

Formal study	In practice	Citizenship
Acquiring additional qualifications as part of a framework of post-registration social work qualification	Taking on additional roles and responsibilities, for example, acting up whilst another is on maternity leave	Active membership of political party/engagement with political challenge
Acquiring education and training in other fields which can be seen to enrich personal practice and contextual awareness	Taking on mentoring and teaching roles in team or service; taking on support of students (for shadowing, as work-based supervisor/practice educator)	Active membership of community-based action group

Taking courses which are not part of a framework of qualification which can be seen to enhance and enrich practice	Contributing to/suggesting research projects/new learning within the workplace	Active support to others
Take responsibility for identifying own learning needs and planning to meet them	Self-leadership through professional conduct	Maintain HCPC standards of ethics in personal conduct and taking opportunities to develop knowledge and skills

Progress Check

The focus of this chapter has direct relevance to Professional Leadership, a discreet domain amongst the nine capabilities required by all registered social workers and described in the Professional Capabilities Framework (PCF) as to:

> take responsibility for the professional learning and development of others through super-vision, mentoring, assessing, research, teaching, leadership and management.
>
> (TCSW, 2012)

As with all PCF domains, professional leadership must be continually demonstrated across a social worker's professional career and what is expected varies depending on the role the social worker occupies.

This chapter has invited the reader to think of themselves as a leader and to review their understanding of what leadership in social work practice is. Following on from this, the reader has also been encouraged to think about when and how they currently exercise leadership. Using Katz's (1955) typology of leadership skills (technical, human and conceptual), the reader might take this opportunity to evaluate their leadership skills with a view to forming a plan for their future development.

Chapter Summary

In this chapter, we have explored why leadership skills are relevant to social workers at every stage in their professional development. Thinking about leadership as an activity which is distributed widely across roles and which is essentially relational in nature, those behaviours which embody and express leadership have been identified. In this way, the approach taken by this chapter has reflected that of the PCF which indicates the importance of leadership at all points in social workers' careers. Specific skills associated with leadership have been discussed and opportunities for skills development have been highlighted. Perhaps ironically, many of the skills of leadership which are often and traditionally linked with senior management roles have been described by theorists and researchers as surprisingly similar to those relational, motivational, responsive and organisational abilities which social workers demonstrate daily.

Further Reading

● McKitterick, B. (2015) *Self-leadership in Social Work: Reflections from Practice*. Bristol: Policy Press.

Written by a social worker and social work manager, this book strongly supports the confident and authoritative leadership of social work practitioners.

● Northouse, P. (2013) *Leadership: Theory and Practice*, 6th edition. London: Sage.

An accessible but detailed introduction of the wide range of leadership theories. The format of the chapters is helpful and keeps the practice manifestations of various approaches very much in mind.

References

Alimo-Metcalf, B. and Alban-Metcalf, J. (2005) Leadership: Time for a New Direction? *Leadership 1* (1): 57–71.

Binney, G. Williams, C. and Wilke, G. (2012) *Living Leadership: A Practical Guide for Ordinary Heroes*, 3rd edition. Harlow: Pearson Education.

Cullen, A.F. (2012) Leaders in Our Own Lives. Suggested Indications for Social Work Leadership from a Study of Social Work Practice in a Palliative Care Setting. *British Journal of Social Work*. 1–18.

Delgardo, R. and Stefancic, J. (2012) *Critical Race Theory: An Introduction*. New York: New York University Press.

Gast, L. and Patmore, A. (2012) *Mastering Approaches to Diversity in Social Work*. London: Jessica Kingsley.

Hafford-Letchfield, T. (2009) Management and Organisations in Social Work, 2nd edition. Exeter: Learning Matters.

Hofstede, G. (2003) *Culture's Consequences: Comparing Values, Behaviors, Institutions and Organizations Across Nations*, 2nd edition. Thousand Oaks, CA: Sage.

Jones, R. (2014) *The Story of Baby P: Setting the Record Straight*. Bristol: Policy Press.

Katz, R. L. (1955). Skills of an effective administrator. *Harvard Business Review*, 33(1), 33–42.

Laming, H. (2009) *The Protection of Children in England*: A Progress Report. London: The Stationery Office.

Lawler, J. (2007) Leadership in Social Work: A Case of Caveat Emptor?, *British Journal of Social Work*, 37: 123–141

Lawler, J. and Bilson, A. (2010) *Social Work Management and Leadership: Managing Complexity with Creativity*. Abingdon: Routledge.

Mantell, A. (2013) *Skills for Social Work Practice*, 2nd edition. London: Sage.

McKitterick, B. (2015) *Self-leadership in Social Work: Reflections from Practice.* Bristol: Policy Press.

Miller, W. R. and Rollnick, S. (2002) *Motivational Interviewing: Preparing People for Change.* New York: The Guilford Press.

Morgan, G. (1997) *Images of Organization.* London: Sage.

Munro, E. (2011) *The Munro Review of Child Protection: A Child-Centred System.* London: Department of Education.

Northouse, P. G. (2013) *Leadership: Theory and Practice.* 6th edition. London: Sage.

The College of Social Work (2012) The Professional Capabilities Framework, available at http://www.tcsw.org.uk/pcfsearch.aspx, accessed 11 March 2015.

The Social Work Task Force (2009) *Building a Safe, Confident Future – The Final Report of the Social Work Task Force.* London: Department for Children, Schools and Families.

Thompson, N. (2011) *Promoting Equality: Challenging Discrimination and Oppression,* 3rd edition. Basingstoke: Palgrave Macmillan.

Trotter, C. (1999) *Working With Involuntary Clients: A Guide to Practice.* London: Sage.

10

SKILLS FOR INTER-PROFESSIONAL SOCIAL WORK PRACTICE

Vivienne Barnes

Introduction

This chapter will begin by considering why specific skills in inter-professional practice are important for social workers, including the requirements in law and policy. It will explore definitions of inter-professional practice and different types of teams in which social workers may be involved, for example those teams where a range of different professionals are located within the same building or agency and those where a range of professionals come together for a specific purpose of working with particular individuals, groups or families. The first section will discuss briefly the dynamics of inter-professional interactions to give a context for the skills social workers need. It will explore the perspectives and language of different professionals, their power relationships, professional boundaries and the limits of confidentiality. This section will also include an overview of inter-professional values and ethics.

A major part of the chapter will be devoted to specific skills that social workers need in this aspect of their work, including communication and information sharing with other professionals and agencies and skills in negotiation. This section will also discuss how to value and utilise the expertise of other professionals whilst maintaining confidence in one's own role. Consideration will be given to the dilemmas of inter-professional working and how to handle difficulties and disagreements. Finally, the chapter will consider the vital role of inter-professional teaching and learning, both at the student stage and in continuing professional development. Throughout, there will be reference to other chapters in this book, where relevant additional detail may be available, for example with regard to legal skills, assessment skills or reflective skills.

Why Develop Inter-professional Practice Skills?

Social Work and Inter-professional Practice: The Context

Social workers find themselves in contact with a range of other professionals and agencies whatever their field of practice might be, including work with children and families, older people, people with disabilities, mental health issues or youth offending. This may be in a range of situations such as making and receiving referrals, attending joint meetings or working together in formal or more informal teams.

Increasingly, inter-professional working is one of the core requirements of professional practice in health, social care and education. The Professional Capabilities Framework (TCSW, 2012) for social work states this clearly, as explored in more detail later in the chapter, and similar emphasis is given to inter-professional working in other professions. For example, the Teachers' Standards (Department for Education, 2011) talk about developing 'effective professional relationships' and 'The Code: Standards of Conduct, Performance and Ethics for Nurses and Midwives' (Nursing and Midwifery Council, 2010) requires that these professionals 'work with others to protect and promote the health and wellbeing of those in your care'.

This emphasis on collaboration between services has grown in the UK since the late 1970s and has gathered momentum. In 1989 the government set out principles for joint financial responsibility between health and social services for community care (Department of Health, 1989) and effective joint working was seen as key. Subsequently, in the field of mental health, collaboration between health services and other relevant agencies aimed to provide more comprehensive care to service users (Department of Health, 1998). New Labour policies drove the agenda further. The integration of services provided to children and families was intended to blur the boundaries of public, private and voluntary agencies by joining these in Children's Trusts. Such 'joined-up' services, reinforced by the Children's Plan (Department for Children Schools and Families, 2007), were considered cost-effective as well as being able to deliver better outcomes for service users. More recently, the Children and Families Act, 2014, has emphasised the need for professionals to work together for disabled children, and in adults' services, one of the main aims of the Health and Social Care Act, 2012, is 'promoting better integration of health and care services'.

The benefits of inter-professional working have been expressed by many writers on the subject (Barrett et al., 2005; Quinney and Hafford-Letchfield, 2012). Banks's (2004: 131) research in a youth offending and community safety

Reflective Exercise 10.1: **Working with a range of professionals**

What are the other professionals and agencies that social workers work with in services for:

　Children?

　Older people?

　Mental health?

Can you think of circumstances where these professionals will need to communicate with social workers about their service users?

service looked at the impact of inter-professional working and the changes it had effected. The study involved professionals from the police, social services, health, education and probation. Despite the acknowledged challenges and differences in the professionals' values and cultures, the research participants considered that there were benefits from inter-professional practice if managed effectively in improved services for service users by the following:

● reducing overlap between services;

● greater consistency and continuity of services;

● improved communication and information sharing between professionals;

● the ability to provide a more 'streamlined' and 'seamless' service.

(Banks, 2004: 131)

Preventing Risk to Service Users

A more detailed discussion of skills in risk assessment is not only found in Chapter 5 but also is discussed briefly here since inter-professional skills are vital in this area of work.

New recruits to the profession are often dismayed by media coverage about social work. The failure of social workers in the UK to share information with other professionals has been repeated in the news and has accounted for many of the recent shifts in policy and law (Munro, 2011). In social work with children and families, numerous child death inquiries (from that of Maria Colwell in 1973 to that of Daniel Pelka in 2013) have highlighted the need for good communication between the professional and agency workers involved in children's lives. The case of baby Peter Connolly's abuse and death in 2007, whilst in the care of his mother and her boyfriend, is an especially tragic instance of the lack of communication between health, social care and police professionals. Lord Laming who conducted the inquiry commented of the professionals involved as follows:

> It is evident that the challenges of working across organisational boundaries continue to pose barriers in practice, and that cooperative efforts are often the first to suffer when services and individuals are under pressure.
>
> (Laming, 2009: 36)

The subsequent practice of creating a 'team around the child' is one that aims to maximise communication and reduce risk to individual children, by placing the child as the central focus of the relevant professionals involved (such as health visitors, teachers, early years workers and police) and promoting 'joined-up working', information sharing and early intervention, all coordinated by a lead professional, usually the social worker (Children's Workforce Development Council, 2009).

Definitions

In the above discussions, you may have noticed several different terms used for inter-professional practice. Terms people use in this context include 'partnership working', 'collaboration', 'inter-agency' and 'multi-professional practice'. Here, we are using an umbrella term 'inter-professional practice' for the sake of simplicity, for as Leathard (2003) says of the many definitions, 'what everyone is really talking about is simply learning and working together' (5). Pollard et al. (2005) note that the prefix *multi* tends to denote the involvement of workers from different agencies but unlike *inter* does not denote collaboration between them (10).

Types of Teams

To add to this complexity, teams may be located in separate agencies and come together to work on individual cases, as with 'teams around the child'. They may be located in the same building but in different parts of it, like a hospital, where for example, doctors, nurses, physiotherapists, occupational therapists and social workers come together to provide a range of specialist care for particular patients. Alternatively, different professionals may work together regularly as an identified team as in community mental health teams where all work together with the majority of their service users. Many of the same issues arise for such 'co-located' teams as for those that come together for an individual case, as may be seen from several research studies described in the following section.

Different Perspectives: Barriers and Supports

Differing Cultures, Identities and Language

Particular professional groups adhere to different basic beliefs, values and norms. For example, a very common one that social workers encounter is the difference between a medical and social model of understanding their service users' lives (Smith, 2008). Social workers often regard the medical model used by health professionals that focuses on the pathology of the individual as an extremely narrow one in relation to their own holistic view of the individual as part of family and societal systems.

Health and social care professionals are socialised into the culture of their chosen profession during their training. They learn their profession's common values and favoured approaches, as well as the preferred language to use (Hall, 2005). Professional codes and standards quoted above, though similar as we have noted in reference to inter-professional practice, are subtly different in their focus.

One of the features of professionals' everyday lives is the specialist language they use, sometimes pejoratively called 'jargon'. In particular, the medical profession uses specialised terms that many others do not understand, but social work also has many of its own. Trethivick (2012) notes that in social care, specialist terms can also be misunderstood by the general public. She cites the Social Services Inspectorate (1991) findings in a survey of service users that terms such as 'agencies' were taken to mean 'second hand clothes shops' and eligibility to mean 'a good marriage catch' (165). Added to these are the acronyms that professionals regularly use such as YOT (Youth Offending Team), CAMHS (Child and Adolescent Mental Health Services) and CP (Child Protection).

Reflective Exercise 10.2: **Specialist language in social work**

Can you think of words used in social work practice that could be misunderstood by other professionals or by service users?

Can you think of any more widely used acronyms and abbreviations in social work in addition to those above?

Professional boundaries and identities can be a hindrance or a help to inter-professional working (Bolin, 2010; Bell and Allain, 2011; Lewin and Reeves, 2011; Rose, 2011). Too strong a professional identity or boundary can weaken people's collaboration and give rise to an 'us and them' mentality. For example, a teacher may insist that education is his remit and may say that he will not consider his students' difficulties in family life, since social workers should be responsible for such wider family matters. Very flexible boundaries may lead to concerns about lack of specialist expertise and what is termed 'hybridisation', creating professionals who are, for example, part-teacher and part-social worker. Jones et al. (2013) use the metaphor of multi-professional teams as 'soups' or 'salads' in their study of professionals' roles in these teams. They describe soups as a blend of professionals where their specialist roles become less distinct (hybrid). Salads, on the other hand, are teams where individual characteristics and contributions remain separate and clearly identifiable.

Interesting research around this area includes Rose's (2011) study of eight inter-professional teams from different areas of children's services. These teams involved a variety of professionals including psychologists, nurses, social workers, teachers, speech therapists and mental health workers. Rose found that there were several dilemmas around the professionals' role identity. The study highlighted the importance of understanding and respecting individuals' roles and their contribution for successful inter-professional working, especially the differences and the overlaps in the professionals' work. Some of the research participants saw it as important to remain allied to their own specialism and keep their expertise, otherwise their identity and their unique contribution within the team became lost and the team might become a 'homogeneous mass' (159). Similarly, Bolin's (2010) research studied social workers and teachers working together in a school in Sweden and identified their negotiation of common and separate 'territories' and the way some workers carefully 'patrolled' the professional boundaries to avoid becoming 'hybrids'. Another, but different, example of resistance to inter-professional working is provided by Lewin and Reeves's (2011) study of health professionals within a large NHS teaching hospital. They found that the formal collaboration mechanisms such as ward rounds and multi-disciplinary team meetings served mainly as window dressing, and the professionals worked largely in parallel. The main inter-professional communications were via unplanned activities such as corridor talk and conversations at patients' bedsides or at the nurses' ward station.

Further challenges to successful inter-professional practice are raised when we consider different professional values.

Values and Ethics

Many commentators and researchers highlight the importance of values and professional ethics in inter-professional working (Hudson, 2002; Banks, 2004; Skaerbaek, 2010). Banks (2004) discusses the view that differing professional values may get in the way of inter-professional collaboration as they may lead to a fundamental lack of mutual understanding. For example, as we shall consider further below, confidentiality may be viewed differently by different professionals. However, Banks (2004) argues that very different perspectives, besides causing disagreements, may also stimulate debates between professionals and this conflict can lead to reflection and renegotiation. Irvine and McPhee (2007) also note this potentially creative element of inter-professional working. They maintain that ethical standpoints in inter-professional working can 'emerge out of actual ongoing deliberation and negotiation between "conversational partners"' and are 'localised in time, space and social power, constituted in the contact zone on the border of professions' (150). Similarly, Skaerbaek (2010) argues that knowledge and ethics in this area are linked, and knowledge needs to be co-creational for better collaboration.

Banks (2010) maintains that we need to think about professional ethics in a new way since this is a time of change in professional life. In traditional professional ethics, distinct professions such as medicine and social work considered their ethical codes in relation to the welfare of their service users only. However, because of the demands of inter-professional working and at a time when service users and carers are also deemed 'experts by experience' (Skilton, 2011), individual workers have complex loyalties and accountabilities. Banks (2010) proposes a more complex model which takes account of ethical relationships with other professionals as well as with service users and where ethical issues need to be negotiated differently. This would be a pluralist, more relational ethical model, one that includes ethics of care and phenomenological and dialogical ethics (as considered in Chapter 3).

Power Dynamics: Whose Reality?

> In the final analysis, power is the right to have your definition of reality prevail over all other people's definition of reality.
>
> (Rowe, 1997: 16)

Hierarchies, professional status and power relationships contribute to the debate about inter-professional practice, as recognised by Hudson (2002), Skaerbaek (2010) and Rose (2011). Although leadership of inter-professional 'teams' may be necessary, sometimes professionals' views may be marginalised by others they work with or not heard at all. Skaerbaek's (2010) study of professionals working together in a 'psychiatric hospital' ward revealed that efforts to enable different professionals to be heard did not necessarily mean that they were listened to but that a medical discourse prevailed over others. Similarly Hudson's (2002) study of GPs, community nurses and social workers working in the community found that professional status was an important factor and GPs tended to assume a leadership role. Whilst finding many barriers to inter-professional working, Hudson nevertheless offers an 'optimistic' model to avoid fragmentation and to deal with increasing policies of co-location. His 'optimistic' ideas based on his research findings can be summarised as follows (16):

- Individual professionals may have more in common with members of a different profession than with members of their own.

- Socialisation to a work group can override hierarchy and professional differences.

- The values of trust and service to service users can promote inter-professional collaboration and professionals can join forces as a collective to achieve goals, including better service delivery and outcomes.

Inter-professional Skills

Communication

The importance of good communication as a social worker is discussed in detail in Chapters 1 and 2. Writers on the topic such as Trethivick (2012) emphasise that clarity of verbal and written communication is just as important when working with other professionals as when working with service users. For example, the skills of active listening apply just as much to practice with other professionals as to work with service users.

> Listening skills are essential in a whole range of different situations, when listening to colleagues, attending meetings, engaging in inter-agency collaboration, in fact in all situations where communication is a central theme.
>
> (Trethivick, 2012: 171)

It is important to listen and to set aside any stereotypes we may have about other professional groups and any pre-judgments about their perspective. For example, in a meeting with other professionals, using open questions and summarising the views of others can assist with the discussion by facilitating a deeper exploration of the issues (Barrett and Keeping, 2005: 21). By doing this we can tune in to any particular concerns they might have about risks to an older person or a child.

It is easy as a social worker to push your professional agenda forward without due consideration of the perspective of the health professional, the teacher or the police officer. Hence it is also important to gain a good understanding of the work of these allied professionals, through networking, discussion and joint training. Even within social work, the perspective of the social worker in a child safeguarding team may well differ from that of the social worker for the child's mother who suffers from mental ill health (see the case study below).

Case Study 10.1: **Irene and Sylvie**

Irene is a 40-year-old woman who has been in hospital several times because she has bipolar disorder. She is the main carer for her daughter, Sylvie, aged six, who has had to move into foster care when her mother has had to go into a mental health unit. On some of the occasions when she has been unwell, Irene has wandered off from the house and left Sylvie on her own.

As the social worker from Children's Services for Sylvie, it is important that you know when Irene is not well so that you can ensure her daughter's safety, but when a social worker from the Community Mental Health Team last visited and Irene's health was deteriorating she did not let you know and there was a crisis in the middle of the night when the police were called by a neighbour.

What steps could you take to try to ensure that there is better communication next time?

Who might you involve in this process?

What kind of communication with those involved might be most effective?

Sharing Information

McCray (2013) helpfully details the past failures of information sharing between professionals, which are summarised here:

- Professionals working in isolation in their own agencies.

- Misplaced concerns about confidentiality.

- Failures in processing information, such as a lack of coordination, not sending correct or clear information and failure to notice or interpret information properly.

- Lack of clarity about roles and responsibilities, poor interpersonal dynamics and stereotyping other professionals thus undermining confidence in their views (132).

There is plenty of government guidance that emphasises the importance of sharing information between professionals. The series of publications that includes 'Information Sharing: Guidance for Practitioners and Managers' (Department for Children Schools and Families, 2008) considers in detail the way professionals should share information in different service settings and between services. It looks at sharing information in preventative work, in service users' transitions between children's and adults' services and where there is risk to a child or an adult. It gives guidance about the limits of information sharing and the laws that govern this. Sharing information is especially vital where risk is involved. As discussed earlier, failures to share information have been reported as contributing to preventable child deaths. The latest guidance for professionals and agencies about safeguarding children and young people, Working Together (2013) says:

> Effective sharing of information between professionals and local agencies is essential for effective identification, assessment and service provision.
>
> (15)

The mechanics of sharing information demands good written and verbal skills as outlined above. Making referrals to other agencies and receiving their details such as the spelling of names, addresses and dates of birth should be accurate and need extreme care. The use of modern technology can aid communication, as in the use of group emails to communicate developments and to consult with a group of professionals involved in work with individual service users.

Confidentiality and Data Protection

Professional ethical codes including social work's HCPC (2012a) Standards of Conduct, Performance and Ethics state, 'You must respect the confidentiality of service users'. However, complete confidentiality may not be possible. How should social workers manage the dilemma of maintaining confidentiality and also sharing information?

There are times when other professionals refuse to share information on the grounds of patient confidentiality. Traditional medical ethics has led to reluctance on the part of some GPs and hospital doctors to share necessary information with social workers, even where there may be an element of risk, because they feel this is breaching confidentiality. The GPs' point of view is documented in a study by Tompsett et al. (2009), while the social workers' view is evident in Barnes's (2013) study with education, social work and health professionals. Several social workers talked about their difficulties in obtaining information from health professionals. One said:

> GPs – it's awful to say – are a dead loss really. You can very rarely get hold of them. When you do get hold of them, they come out with all this withholding of information.

In such circumstances, social workers may need to explain the duties involved in safeguarding adults and children that override such concerns for the sake of safety.

The Data Protection Act 1998 requires social workers and other professionals to keep personal information and records safe and only to share those with the individual's consent, except where there are identified safeguarding issues. There are questions about whether sharing information may infringe the privacy of family life. Munro (2007) discusses this dilemma in social work and, whilst recognising the protective function of confidentiality, questions whether this erosion of privacy may lead to unhelpful state intrusion and control.

Negotiation and Conflict

Negotiation is an important skill in inter-professional practice, in terms of reaching shared understandings with other professionals. Shared agreement requires some flexibility of all parties and a willingness to compromise. Key to this is understanding the underlying thinking of the other person (Lishman, 2009). If, for example, a health visitor is unhappy with the standard of hygiene in a family where there are young children, and you, as the social worker, think it is adequate, it will be important to discuss together how you have both reached a different judgement. It may be that the health visitor has more knowledge of the health risks involved or judgements may be based on norms arrived at through your respective training or your personal upbringing. Where there remains disagreement, it is still important to respect the other's point of view.

Part of negotiating is being clear about one's own professional starting point so that other professionals can understand the values and perspectives we have. Other professionals may have a different viewpoint because of their role, as discussed above, or there may be pressure within their organisation because of management restriction on resources. Where there appears to be an injustice, for example, in withholding resources, it may be the role of a social worker to challenge this. As such this is allied to the advocate's role. Here, different skills, those of presenting a case clearly and rallying support from others, such as your manager, may help. You may also need to find out where the actual or potential block exists. It may not be the front-line professional such as a teacher or community nurse you are dealing with. It could be someone in a management role, for example, in their organisation who is constraining support or resources. You may need to persist in the face of conflict and initial failure.

Shell (2006) explores different styles and stages of negotiation. He explains the importance of proper preparation for this: not only being armed with factual information but also being aware of one's own values and those of others. The next stage is exchanging information and asking questions, before actually trying to 'bargain'. At this point, there will often be some elements of compromise followed by clear conclusions and agreed actions. Styles of negotiation mentioned by Shell are summarised as follows:

- Competing – this style is about a drive to *win* that overrides all other considerations and may point to some inflexibility and even insecurity in considering others' views.

- Avoiding – this is where people avoid conflict, favouring the maintenance of a positive relationship.

- Accommodating and compromising – these may give too much value to relationships with others, and compromises can be made too easily. However, compromisers may be helpful in reaching some form of agreement.

- Collaborating – this involves some empathy with others' viewpoints and an attempt at consensus, but this may not always be achievable.

Case Study 10.2: **Lorna**

Lorna is 20 and is about to have her first baby. There were concerns about whether she would be able to care for the baby as she was suffering from severe depression just a year ago. Lorna spent years in a range of residential and foster homes during her childhood. She will have to leave her semi-independent living accommodation which was provided by social services because they are unable to provide for young mothers.

The local housing department have refused to provide social housing for Lorna and her baby as she has rent arrears of around £100. The leaving care team say that they are only able to assist with providing accommodation until she is 21 – just before the baby is born.

As the social worker for the unborn baby, you want to help negotiate for Lorna and her baby to have a settled place to live. You are aware that, as a young care leaver, she has the right to be afforded priority for social housing.

> Think about your preferred negotiating style (of those listed above). You may wish to think about how you handled a recent situation where you have had to negotiate.
>
> In negotiating with staff from the housing department and from the leaving care team, what might be the effect of using your preferred style?
>
> Could you usefully change to a different style? What effect might this have had?

Smethurst and Long (2013) point out that negotiating, especially where there are conflicting views, can give rise to strong emotions and that it is wise to be aware of one's anger, anxiety or frustration.

Handling Conflicts

Moving on logically from negotiation, we look at the inevitable conflicts that may and do arise in inter-professional working. In Barnes's (2013) research, the professionals from education, health and social work talked far more about the conflicts than about the successes of working together. In relation to profession-als' conflicts, emotions can be highly charged. Sometimes conflict can be hidden rather than overt, and professionals may seethe without being open about this. Conflict may also lead to avoidance. Ground rules in teams or meet-ings where conflict is expected may be helpful, by having rules, for example, that only one person may speak at a time, requiring honesty in feedback to ideas and by recognising that there could be a number of solutions possible and that these should be explored (Barrett and Keeping, 2005: 24).

Professional Identity and Role

This section on the development of one's professional identity and role is linked to the above discussion of research about differing professional cultures, identi-ties and language. It will take a student or a newly qualified worker some time to understand the boundaries of their role in whichever setting they are working. This confidence in one's role is a gradual process built up through feedback from supervisors and colleagues as well as critical reflection (see Chapter 8). How do we gain an understanding of the roles of other professionals and how do we expect them to be able to understand ours? This is particularly problematic, as Barrett and Keeping (2005) point out, in services that are constantly changing through changes in laws and policies. Besides, some roles may be blurred and overlapping. For example, in community mental health teams, it may be a com-munity nurse or a social worker who conducts an assessment. The use of a Single Assessment Process (SAP) in adult care is another example of this in which differ-ent professionals use the same assessment tool. Learning about the work of other professionals is a process that evolves through working together, through training and later as a qualified social worker, as discussed at the end of this chapter.

A related area in inter-professional working, and a positive one, is being able to draw on the expertise of other professionals. Critically, this involves some understanding of their role and relies on trust and building good individual rela-tionships with other professionals. In Barnes's (2013) study, professionals emphasised the importance of these individual relationships and of creating professional networks. One social worker talked about the benefits of each draw-ing on the other's expertise in her work with a head teacher and commented:

> That type of working relationship is just brilliant because you've got someone there that's got twenty years of teaching experience, five years of being a head teacher.

That person is an expert in education – so why am I trawling through the internet, trying to get information that I could probably get in thirty seconds from her? And having that is really good.

Conversely, how do we know the limits of our expertise? It can be unhelpful and even dangerous for service users if we try to work beyond our capacity. This is especially tempting when resources are in short supply. A children's social worker, for example, may attempt specialist work with a young person who has suffered sexual abuse if they find there are no immediately available specialist counselling services for children in their area. If they have not had proper training, this can result in more damage to the young person than benefit. In such cases, it may be better to wait until a resource becomes available or to seek resources for appropriate counselling services more widely.

Progress Check

Inter-professional practice requires capabilities within all the domains of the Professional Capabilities Framework (PCF) at registered social worker level but a key one within the domain 'Contexts and Organisations' is:

> Take an active role in inter-professional and inter-agency work, building own network and collaborative working (8.7).

The social worker quoted above highlights some of the benefits for a qualified worker of inter-professional collaboration with a head teacher, but from the beginning of a student's practice experience, it is important to build up knowledge of the roles of other professionals and to develop one's own professional identity.

Another key issue in inter-professional working is highlighted in the section above on 'Communication' and this is emphasised in the HCPC Standards of Proficiency (SoP):

> Be able to engage in inter-professional and inter-agency communication (8.9).

As remarked earlier, this involves learning to listen with respect and to avoid stereotyping other professionals. It also requires a commitment to sharing information where appropriate and to learning about the boundaries of confidentiality.

Inter-professional Teaching and Learning

A good foundation of inter-professional working should be a part of teaching and learning at all stages of a social worker's career. In Higher Education, this could mean studying modules alongside other professionals in training such as nurses, occupational therapists and teachers. Critics, however, have pointed out that teaching staff need to be aware that merely placing students from different student professional groups together does not necessarily lead to optimum understanding and can even lead to conflict between the students. As Hean et al. (2006) have found, many social work students arrive at their courses with already well-developed ideas about allied professionals in health and social care which may influence their learning (162).

The UK Centre for the Advancement of Inter-professional Education (www. caipe.org.uk) defines two types of student inter-professional learning and are as follows:

- multi-professional education that involves different professionals learning side by side;

- inter-professional education that involves different professionals learning about each other and learning to collaborate effectively for the benefit of service users.

Most social work practice placements provide useful opportunities for inter-professional work and this can be maximised through good planning and understanding of the importance of this by Practice Educators. Students may be involved in shadowing other professionals, joint working, specialist teams and so on, and it is helpful to reflect on learning during these situations.

Continuous professional development is a requirement of the professional body (HCPC, 2012b). All through a social worker's career, opportunities for joint professional training should arise and it is important to take advantage of these.

Conclusion

- Social workers are required by law, policy and by their professional council (HCPC) to have a good understanding of, and skills in, inter-professional working.

- Research has shown the importance of understanding different professional cultures, roles and values of allied professionals, as well as the effects of power relationships in inter-professional teams.

- Development of communication and negotiation skills is central to good inter-professional practice to promote collaboration and deal with conflicts.

- Social workers need to reflect on the balance between confidentiality and information sharing and the relevance of these to safeguarding service users.

- Learning to collaborate and learning alongside other professionals is an important part of initial training and continuing professional development and is key in the development of professional identity.

Chapter Summary

In this chapter we have considered the nature of inter-professional practice and its relevance to social work. We have explored some of the issues involved in the development and definition of inter-professional practice and research evidence about differing professional cultures, values and boundaries. The main focus of the chapter has been the development of inter-professional skills in social work, examining in detail communication and negotiation skills and inter-professional practice dilemmas.

Further Reading

- Mantell, A. (ed.) (2013) *Skills for Social Work Practice*, 2nd edition. London: Sage/ Learning Matters.

  Contains useful chapters on inter-professional working that provide an overview of collaborative skills and negotiating skills.

- Quinney, A. and Hafford-Letchfield, T. (2012) *Interprofessional Social Work: Effective Collaborative Approaches*, 2nd edition. London: Sage.

  Looks at inter-professional working in different contexts such as youth work, health, justice and education.

- Reeves, S., Lewin, S., Espin, S. and Zwarenstein, M. (2010) *Interprofessional Teamwork for Health and Social Care*. Chichester: WileyBlackwell.

  Examines the theory and practice of effective teams, taking a wide perspective by considering teamwork around the globe.

The *Journal of Inter-professional Care* is a useful peer-reviewed journal that provides a forum for papers about the latest research and theory about inter-professional practice, including health, education and social work.

The website of the UK Centre for the Advancement of Inter-Professional Education contains a variety of learning resources, including publications and multimedia which are free to download. Available at www.caipe.org.uk.

References

Banks, S. (2004) *Ethics, Accountability and the Social Professions*. Basingstoke: Palgrave Macmillan.

Banks, S. (2010) Interprofessional Ethics: A Developing Field? Notes from the *Ethics and Social Welfare* Conference, Sheffield, UK, May, 2010, *Ethics and Social Welfare*, 4 (3): 280–294.

Barnes, V. (2013) *Inter-professional Ethics and Professionals' Attitudes to Children and Young People*. Kingston University: Institute of Child Centred Inter-professional Practice.

Barrett, G. and Keeping, C. (2005) The Processes Required for Effective Inter-professional Working. In Barrett, G., Sellman, D. and Thomas, J. (eds), *Inter-professional Working in Health and Social Care*. Basingstoke: Palgrave Macmillan.

Barrett, G. Sellman, D. and Thomas, J. (eds) (2005) *Inter-professional Working in Health and Social Care*. Basingstoke: Palgrave Macmillan.

Bell, L. and Allain, L. (2011) Exploring Professional Stereotypes and Learning for Inter-professional Practice: An Example from UK Qualifying Level Social Work Education. *Social Work Education*, 30 (3): 266–280.

Bolin, A. (2010) Inter-professional Collaboration Around Children at Risk: A Negotiated Social Order. Paper Presented at 2010 Joint World Conference on Social Work and Social Development: The Agenda, Hong Kong, 11–14 June.

Children's Workforce Development Council (2009) Available at http://webarchive. nationalarchives.gov.uk/20130401151715/https://www.education.gov.uk/publications/ eOrderingDownload/LeadPro_Managers-Guide.pdf, accessed 10 May 2014.

Department for Children, Schools and Families (2007) *The Children's Plan Building Brighter Futures*. London: TSO.

Department for Children Schools and Families (2008) *Information Sharing: Guidance for Practitioners and Managers*. London: TSO.

Department for Education (2011) *The Teachers' Standards*. London: TSO.

Department of Health (1989) *Caring for People: Community Care in the Next Decade and Beyond*. London: HMSO.

Department of Health (1998) *Modernising Mental Health Services: Safe, Sound and Supportive*. London: DOH.

Hall, P. (2005) Interprofessional Teamwork: Professional Cultures as Barriers, *Journal of Interprofessional Care*, 19 (1): 188–196.

Health and Care Professions Council (2012a) *Standards of Conduct, Performance and Ethics*. London: HCPC.

Health and Care Professions Council (2012b) *Your Guide to Our Standards for Continuing Professional Development*. London: HCPC

Hean, S., Macleod Clark, J., Adams, K. and Humphries, D. (2006) Will Opposites Attract? Similarities and Differences in Students' Perceptions of Stereotype Profiles of Other Health and Social Care Professional Groups, *Journal of Inter-professional Care*, 20 (2): 162–181.

Hudson, B. (2002) Interprofessionality in Health and Social Care: The Achilles Heel of Partnership? *Journal of Interprofessional Care*, 16 (1): 7–17.

Irvine, R. and McPhee, J. (2007) Multi-disciplinary Team practice. In Leathard, A. and McLaren, S. (eds), *Ethics: Contemporary Challenges in Health and Social Care*. Bristol: Policy Press.

Jones, R., Bhanbhro, S. M., Grant, R. and Hood, R. (2013) The Definition and Deployment of Differential Core Professional Competencies and Characteristics in Multiprofessional Health and Social Care Teams, *Health and Social Care*, 21 (1): 47–58.

Laming, H. (2009) *The Protection of Children in England: A Progress Report*. London: The Stationery Office.

Leathard, A. (ed.) (2003) *Interprofessional Collaboration: From Policy to Practice in Health and Social Care*. Hove: Routledge.

Lewin, S. and Reeves, S. (2011) Enacting 'team' and 'teamwork': Using Goffman's Theory of Impression Management to Illuminate Interprofessional Practice on Hospital Wards, *Social Science and Medicine, 72* (10): 1595–1602.

Lishman, J. (2009) Personal and Professional Development. In Adams, R., Dominelli, L. and Payne, M. (eds), *Social Work: Themes, Issues and Critical Debates*, 3rd edition. Basingstoke: Palgrave Macmillan.

McCray, J. (2013) Skills for Collaborative Working. In Mantell, A. (ed.), *Skills for Social Work Practice*, 2nd edition. London: Sage/Learning Matters.

Munro, E. (2007) Confidentiality in a Preventive Child Welfare System, *Ethics and Social Welfare*, 1 (1): 41–55.

Munro, E. (2011) *The Munro Review of Child Protection: Final Report. A Child-centred System*. London: TSO.

Nursing and Midwifery Council (2010) *The Code: Standards of Conduct, Performance and Ethics for Nurses and Midwives*. London: NMC.

Pollard, K., Sellman, D. and Senior, B. (2005) The Need for Interprofessional Working. In Barrett, G., Sellman, D. and Thomas. J. (eds), *Inter-professional Working in Health and Social Care*. Basingstoke: Palgrave Macmillan

Quinney, A. and Hafford-Letchfield, T. (2012) *Interprofessional Social Work: Effective Collaborative Approaches*, 2nd edition. London: Sage.

Rose, J. (2011) Dilemmas of Inter-professional Collaboration: Can They Be Resolved? *Children and Society*, 25: 151–163.

Rowe, D. (1997) Foreword in *J. Masson Against Therapy*. Hammersmith: HarperCollins.

Shell, R. (2006) *Bargaining for Advantage: Negotiating Strategies for Reasonable People*. New York: Penguin Books.

Skaerbaek, E. (2010) Undressing the Emperor? On the Ethical Dilemmas of Hierarchical Knowledge, *Journal of Interprofessional Care*, 24 (5): 579–586.

Skilton, C. J. (2011) Involving Experts by Experience in Assessing Students' Readiness to Practice: The Value of Experiential Learning in Student Reflection and Preparation for Practice, *Social Work Education*, 30 (3): 299–311.

Smethurst, C. and Long, R. (2013) Negotiation Skills. In Mantell, A. (ed.), *Skills for Social Work Practice*, 2nd edition. London: Sage/Learning Matters.

Smith, S. (2008) Social Justice and Disability: Competing Interpretations of the Medical and Social Models. In Kristiansen, K., Vehmas, S. and Shakespeare, T. (eds), *Arguing About Disability*. Abingdon: Routledge.

The College of Social Work (2012) Available at http://www.tcsw.org.uk/pcf.aspx, accessed 15 June 2014.

Tompsett, H., Ashworth, M., Atkins, C., Bell, L., Gallagher, A., Morgan, M. and Wainwright, P. (2009). The Child, the Family and the GP: Tensions and Conflicts of Interest in Safeguarding Children, *DCSF Executive Summary DCSF-RBX-09-05-ES*. DCSF: London.

Trethivick, P. (2012) *Social Work Skills and Knowledge*, 3rd edition. Maidenhead: Open University.

11

WORKING WITH RESISTANCE

Elaine Gaskell-Mew and Jane Lindsay

Introduction

Professional social work requires social workers to take an authoritative stance to ensure the survival, safety and well-being of children and adults at risk in our society. Frequently, the people with whom social workers are working do not seek social work services; they are sometimes termed 'involuntary service users' and they may resist social work involvement. Working with resistance and conflict is a routine part of social work practice. Social workers need to develop and maintain robust skills and strategies in order to be able to manage conflict and practise effectively and safely. This chapter explores the following:

1   What is resistance? Defining the concept of resistance in the context of situations where social workers may perceive or experience resistance from service users and carers.

2   What causes resistance? Theoretical perspectives to assist understanding in situations where resistance is encountered.

3   How to work positively with resistance. Providing practical suggestions for social work practice to improve outcomes for service users and carers and to promote service user and practitioner resilience.

What is 'Resistance'?

The *Oxford English Dictionary* (2013) defines resistance in a number of different ways, two of which can be observed in the dynamics between social workers and the users (or 'refusers') of their services:

(i) refusal to accept or comply;

(ii) the use of violence or force to oppose someone or something.

Refusal to Accept or Comply

This may take the form of avoidance such as service users repeatedly failing to keep appointments, being absent from their homes at times of arranged visits or failing to attend meetings. If a social worker feels a rush of relief when the service user fails to answer their door, this feeling should instantly be regarded as a signal to pay particular attention. Ward (2010) in a discussion of the 'use of self' in relationship-based practice points out that vague emotional discomfort can be a raw form of information to be unravelled and scrutinised for significance.

Some service users may keep appointments and accept visits yet still refuse to comply, for example by diverting the social worker's attention from key issues or by withholding relevant information. Some service users or carers may appear to engage when in reality there is only 'disguised compliance'; this term is attributed to Reder et al. (1993) who first described the phenomenon as it emerged from their detailed analysis of 35 child deaths:

> Sometimes, during cycles of intermittent closure, a professional worker would decide to adopt a more controlling stance. However, this was defused by apparent co-operation from the family. We have called this disguised compliance because its effect was to neutralize the professional's authority and return the relationship to closure and the previous status quo.
>
> (Reder et al., 1993: 106–107)

Examples of disguised compliance might include a sudden increase in school attendance, keeping a run of medical appointments or engaging with selected professionals for a limited period of time. A case example is that of 17-month-old Peter Connolly whose mother engaged with social workers in some contexts, for example, regularly attending parenting classes. However, she was dishonest about the cause of Peter's multiple injuries, on one occasion disguising them by smearing chocolate over his face. She also concealed from professionals the presence in her household of her violent partner who was later convicted, jointly with her, of causing Peter's death (Haringey LSCB, 2009).

The Use of Violence or Force to Oppose Someone or Something

There are times when service users may resort to physical force, aggression or believable threats to stop or impede a social worker carrying out their duties. Brandon et al.'s (2009) analysis of 200 serious case reviews reveals significant evidence of social workers failure to assess risk correctly due to intimidation by hostile service users/carers.

Laird (2013) provides a comprehensive analysis of a broad range of recent research data from Australia, the USA and the UK:

> Treated cross-nationally, these studies suggest that 10–20 per cent of all social workers experience some form of physical violence, while 30–60 per cent of them are threatened. Around 60 per cent of all social workers and nearly 100 per cent of child protection workers are subjected to verbal abuse by a service user, parent or other family member.
>
> (Laird, 2013: 2)

Research reviewed by Littlechild (2005) into the effects of service user hostility towards child protection social workers in England and Finland found that physical violence towards social workers is relatively rare and most frequently perpetrated spontaneously by female service users in crisis situations. The gender differentiation is likely, in part anyway, to be because mothers have more face to face contact with social workers than fathers. Littlechild also noted that the power of the social worker in a child protection role may not only 'provoke aggression' but also 'protect' the social worker from more serious attack.

Littlechild's analysis revealed that social workers tended to report physical assaults (though by no means always) and usually received a supportive response from managers when they did. However, they were much less likely to report the menacing 'power and control tactics' which were more often perpetrated by men such as threats of violence to social workers and their families, stalking behaviours and relentless complaints and legal challenges. These behaviours were much more prevalent than physical assaults and had a detrimental effect on social workers' well-being and the quality of their assessments (Littlechild, 2005).

Failure to report psychological abuse can leave social workers at risk of becoming isolated. Smith (2005) warns of the negative consequences of underestimating the impact of fear on the quality of social workers assessments. Stanley and Goddard (2002) in a study of the impact of a long-term aggression from service users likened social workers' responses to that of hostages presenting with 'Stockholm Syndrome'. This phenomenon was first noted in the 1970s during a situation when hostages refused to give evidence against their captors following their release. A key feature of the syndrome is the isolation of the victim leading to their alignment with the perpetrator's perspective as a means of self-defence. There are clear implications here regarding the need for supportive supervision of social workers who are facing hostility and threats.

Laird (2013: 9) highlights the problems arising from 'role incompatibility' between care and control functions in the safeguarding role. Taylor (2011) writes about the ethical dilemma of 'working together' with parents in keeping with government policies (HM Gov, 2013) while conducting investigatory activities such as asking to look into bedrooms or food cupboards or making unannounced visits (Taylor, 2011: 89). Sir Martin Narey, in his independent review of the education of children's social workers, comments that too much attention may have been given to teaching empowering and collaborative working skills and that:

> There is no acknowledgement that when one is protecting the interests of a neglected or abused child, there are very real limits on the extent to which working in partnership is appropriate. (Narey, 2014: 8)

This critical 'dilemma' will be revisited later in this chapter.

What Causes Resistance?

Some Examples with Reference to a Range of Theoretical Perspectives are Explored Below.

It is vital for social workers to be self-aware regarding their theoretical understanding of resistance as this will influence how they interpret service users' intentions and how they then respond to service users' behaviour.

Service users/carers may genuinely regard their behaviour as normal and hence resent the intrusion of professional intervention in their lives.

A social learning theory approach, originally attributed to Bandura (1977), might explain resistance to change in terms of the difficulty of challenging deeply embedded, learned behaviours, cultural values and beliefs, for example regarding the use of corporal punishment or matters of appropriate physical intimacy in relation to children and partners. Renteln (2010) provides a comprehensive discussion with real case examples from American courts where the defence of 'different cultural values' has been used to mitigate for defendants facing charges of child abuse. Phillips (2010) provides a discussion pertaining to English law including the example below,

> where a Nigerian mother was prosecuted for the ceremonial scarring of the cheeks of her nine and fourteen year old sons. In this case, the fact that the scarification would have been accepted as a normal part of Yoruba custom, and that the Nigerian community in Britain was probably not aware that the practice was contrary to English law, was felt to change the status of the offence ... [The mother] was nonetheless convicted: in English criminal law, a minority custom cannot be a defence to a prosecution, unless this is explicitly allowed for in legislation. She was, however, given an absolute discharge.
>
> (Phillips, 2010: 85)

The difficulties of challenging deeply embedded culturally acceptable abuse can be seen in the practice of female genital mutilation (removal by 'cutting' away some or all of a female's external genitalia, often without anaesthetic, usually during her childhood or infancy). Mason (2014) reported that 'not a single case has been brought to the British courts since specific laws against FGM were introduced in 1983 and 2002' (Mason 2014: 14).

A cognitive behavioural approach may explain a service user's values as 'distorted beliefs' driving problematic behaviours thus rendering those beliefs appropriate targets for therapeutic intervention (Sheldon in Stepney and Ford, 2000). For example, a parent's 'belief' that insulting children by calling them stupid, ungrateful or lazy will motivate them to behave well could be explored as part of a parenting programme (Scott, 2010).

Issues relating to values, beliefs and diversity will often create powerful feelings and challenging dynamics. Social workers may sometimes misuse their professional power based upon negative interpretations and stereotyping of service users' values and behaviour. Conversely they may avoid exploring important information for fear of 'getting it wrong' and causing unintentional offence (Gast and Patmore, 2012). Lord Laming's report into the death of eight-year-old Victoria Climbié, who died following months of torture by her aunt and her aunt's male partner, noted that social workers' assumptions around racial difference had a role to play in the misinterpretation of important information relating to assessment of Victoria's behaviour and her injuries (Laming, 2003: 345–346).

In a skills-deficit approach, the service user may be perceived as having a lack of learned skills and understanding about what children need to thrive, leading to a 'failure of parenting capacity'(Cleaver et al., 2011). Thus a person's ability to nurture a child (or care for an adult at risk) can be compromised by trauma or neglect in their own infancy.

Although young children are very resilient, their coping mechanisms, for example closing off emotional pain, can ultimately lead to maladapted attachment styles and poor emotional management in adulthood (Howe, 1995).

> Attachment theory is probably the most helpful and understandable theoretical model. Insecure or poor attachments, together with experiences of trauma, tend to lead to difficulties in
>
> • accurately interpreting the thoughts and feelings of others and
> • managing relationships, which trigger strong and unmanageable emotions.
>
> (Craissati et al., 2011: 21)

Extreme psychological and physical abuse of the child may even result in delayed brain development (Perry, 2005) or the individual developing a personality disorder in adulthood. Here is a succinct description of anti-social personality disorder:

● highly resistant and resentful of control or domination by others;

● prone to aggression at the level of physical fights/assaults;

● deceitfulness, such as conning, repeated lying and use of aliases for personal gain;

- reckless disregard for the safety of self and others;

- competitive, blunt, intimidating;

- unremorseful for hurting others'.
                              (NHS Camden and Islington Impact Team, 2012: 1)

There are elements in this description which clearly overlap with some of the most challenging behaviours displayed by the minority of service users considered to be the most dangerous and resistant in high-risk social work situations. It is virtually inevitable that social workers will find themselves working with individuals who have a personality disorder at some stage. It may help to foster compassion by understanding that personality disorder in an adult is often the result of a traumatic infancy. One of the many failings highlighted in the death of baby Peter Connolly was that his mother's own disturbed childhood was not sufficiently explored (Haringey LSCB, 2009).

Service users may have a long history of social work involvement with little experience of positive outcomes. In some cases, service users may have had negative prior experiences of intervention, for example mothers who are victims of domestic abuse may be called to account, by a host of professionals, for their inability to protect their children, without any perceived increase in protection for themselves from their abuser. See Hester (2011) for a discussion of the complexities and contradictions facing abused women by the demands of different professional systems intervening in their lives.

Service users may associate professional intervention with previous negative experiences of authority, for example a service user may have survived traumatic experiences in the education system resulting in powerful feelings of fear and humiliation. A psycho-social approach (Kenny and Kenny, 2000) might explain this service user's resistance to intervention in terms of their unconscious transference of negative feelings from past experiences. In a cognitive-behavioural interpretation, this service user's resistance may be viewed as the generalisation of a specific fear (Sheldon, 2000). In either interpretation, the social worker has the task of creating a positive experience of authority and restoring lost trust.

Prospective service users may face complex dilemmas about the unwanted consequences of seeking social work involvement; for example struggling parents may fear losing custody or access to their children, or for older people, there may be the fear of losing their rights to live in their own homes, for children of abusive parents, the fear of never seeing their parents again. People with disabilities who are being abused by a family carer or partner may fear losing the only person with whom they feel they could have a close relationship and a life lived in their own home (LGA, 2013).

There is arguably an inevitable level of 'shame' or embarrassment attached to the notion of failing to cope 'socially' without professional support in our society which overtly values and rewards individual achievement (Gast and Patmore, 2012). When recruiting low-income families into parenting programmes, Webster-Stratton found that parents were best persuaded to attend sessions by 'selling' the programme as something to help with their child's education rather than their own parenting capacity (Smith, 2011). McNeill's work with desistance from offending behaviour has revealed the significance of creating, and sustaining, a positive identity as one of the key components for effecting a lasting change in behaviour (McNeill, 2009).

Service users whose lives are dominated by substance abuse may struggle to contend with both the shame of being labelled as an 'addict' and the consequences of any service provision which threatens to deprive them of their drug of choice even though using this substance may threaten everything they care about. Understanding addiction can impact on professional value judgements such as how a social worker views a mother who prioritises buying cigarettes above buying fresh fruit for her child.

Prochaska and Di Clemente's observations, arising from work with people with substance abuse problems, highlight the crucial importance of recognising that change is a dynamic process with recognisable stages and that any attempt to force people to change before they are ready will meet with resistance. The stages are 'pre-contemplation' where there may be no recognition of a problem and certainly no consideration of change to 'contemplation' (recognising the problem and considering change) followed by 'preparation' (getting ready to change), 'action' (making the change) and 'maintenance' (keeping it up). There may be periods of lapse and relapse before change is fully achieved. Each of these distinct stages produces characteristic language and behaviours, described as 'change talk' and behaviours which sustain or undermine change. If social workers understand and recognise these stages, they will assess motivation more accurately and thus avoid creating more resistance (Prochaska and Di Clemente, 2005).

A minority of service users with mental health issues may have powerfully destructive tendencies which threaten their own safety and that of their families and others. Brandon et al. (2009) present evidence to support the correlation between poor mental health of a parent and increased severity of abuse and neglect of a child. A specialist mental health social worker has the role of upholding the rights of the service user in the face of a potentially oppressive medical diagnosis and the power to support or veto a compulsory admission to a secure treatment environment (Mental Health Act, 2007). This powerful role may attract equally powerful responses from service users, including resistance and refusal to engage. It is vitally important for all social workers to be aware of information from multi-agency sources pertaining to mental health issues suffered by people they are working with.

Service users who have been convicted of criminal offences may have similar needs to many social work service users and are often the very same people. People subject to compulsory supervision are often resentful towards figures of authority:

> Offenders subject to community supervision have very high levels of need. This means that, in addition to addressing their client's offending behaviour, practitioners often have to deal with problems relating to poor parenting, abuse, neglect, and damaged relationships, criminal and anti-social peers, low educational attainment, substance abuse or dependency, high levels of impulsiveness and aggressiveness, poverty, poor housing and/or homelessness. Irrespective of how these difficulties are related to offending behaviour, they have important implications for supervision and the skills required to prompt and support reductions in re-offending.
>
> (McNeill et al., 2005: 12)

Service users may be resistant to engage due to overwhelming practical obstacles such as transport costs and child-care difficulties (Smith et al. 2011). Social workers coming from a psychodynamic perspective might interpret such behaviour as a 'defence mechanism' whereby the service user is seen as unable to deal with his or her emotions and unconsciously constructing obstacles (Kenny and Kenny, 2000). However, it may be that practical obstacles simply outweigh the perceived benefits for the service user at the time of the intervention (Smith et al., 2012).

Service users may resist engagement in group interventions when there is an under-representation of particular groups. Examples might include fathers in parenting programmes or minority ethnic service users (DCSF, 2007). Social workers may interpret the failure of a father to attend meetings as a lack of commitment when actually the father is feeling isolated, judged and generally excluded by services which have little expectation or provision for engaging men (YJB, 2011).

Service users fear that social work intervention will place them at higher risk of harm. Unfortunately, this is sometimes true, for example in cases of domestic abuse where a woman may be ordered to separate from her abusive partner. If there is no professional engagement with the man (perhaps because he behaves aggressively or because of erroneous assumptions that risk is reduced simply because he has left the home), the woman and her children may be placed at even higher risk of harm (Stanley, 2011). There is a growing awareness of the importance of positively engaging with abusive fathers in order to protect women and children (Scott, 2010). It is critically important for social workers to understand the particular dynamics of domestic abuse (Stanley, 2011) and 'so called honour' crime (Stobart, 2009); if unsure of how to proceed they should seek supervision and/or contact specialist agencies for advice.

Social workers are cautioned by Monds-Watson (2011) to remember that everyone has defence mechanisms such as denial, rationalisation and repression at various times and it can be a 'useful defence mechanism' for a social worker to blame service user resistance for an ineffective intervention which may itself be driving the service user away (Monds-Watson in Taylor, 2011: 33).

How to Work Positively with Resistance

It is important for social workers to have a broad understanding of the diversity of causation to inform their decision making and appropriate use of their professional power. Whether resistance is underpinned by a service user's realistic anxieties, their paralysing shame or their manipulative hostility, it is never easy to deal with; if it were easy then this recurring problem would have been resolved before now. The organisation and resourcing of systems of service delivery can have a critical impact on social workers' ability to assess need and risk. In the wake of the Munro analysis of child protection services, there are various systemic service delivery models evolving, which are designed to enhance shared professional decision making and reduce worker isolation and the potential for individual errors (Munro, 2010). So, in light of the evidence reviewed so far, are there any particularly important practice skills which social workers need to develop to enhance safer practice?

Most practitioners who have worked in social work for a number of years will have known a range of colleagues whose practice style may be considered along a continuum. At one extreme are those colleagues renowned for their ability to connect with and relate positively to a wide range of service users, even those who are presenting as very angry or distressed. These colleagues often have good relationships with their peers and managers and appear to be resilient, assertive and emotionally grounded. At the other extreme are colleagues who seem actively to 'wind people up', who frequently hold broadly negative opinions of service users and who may be anxious and filled with resentment about the demands of the work. The difference between the two ends of this continuum cannot be attributed to a particular theoretical model of intervention but arguably to an overarching set of communication skills which will be explored in the following section. The case study below (part 1) relates to some of the issues discussed above and poses questions to be considered in context.

Case Study 11:1 **Lena and her family (part 1)**

Lena is a 14-year-old girl who has lived with her adopted parents Jon and Mel since she was 18 months old. She has two siblings: Alex 12 and Robin ten, also adopted. All three children have ongoing educational and developmental issues. Lena has received social

▶

work and children's mental health services input for many years; she has a history of self-harming, problematic behaviour at school and home and has recently assaulted her adopted mother. Lena is now asking to leave home. Sandra, who qualified as a social worker 12 months previously, works in the child protection team and is allocated the case. Sandra is a mature woman with a previous professional career.

Sandra visits the family at home; Jon and Mel are well-educated professionals; Jon in particular is a high-earning, high-profile individual. The home is immaculate and luxurious. Both parents present as articulate, calm and united despite the current difficulties. Lena is described by them as having emotional and psychological issues due to her traumatic infancy and her biological mother's substance abuse. Sandra, who is of similar age, race and class as Mel, feels some affinity towards her. Mel explains that she 'hate[s] social workers' but understands that they 'need to be seen to do something' so she will engage with Sandra. Sandra thanks Mel for her honesty and her willingness to engage.

Sandra speaks to Lena separately. Lena describes a history of protracted arguments with her mother involving punitive sanctions for apparently petty misdemeanours. Lena tells Sandra that she fears she will do something really bad to herself or her mother if things don't change.

Sandra suggests a course of action to improve the dynamics between Lena and her mother, for example establishing some clear and reasonable boundaries and using praise for good behaviour. Mel agrees to comply but in fact never actually changes her behaviour; she explains her inertia by blaming Lena. Both parents minimise the details of Lena's violence and the risks of physical and emotional harm to Mel and the other children. Sandra continues to develop a trusting relationship with Lena in their individual meetings. Sandra concludes that Lena's mother is emotionally abusive and that there is an imminent risk of serious violence from Lena.

Sandra discusses the case in supervision and a decision is made that Lena should be given the opportunity to live separately from her adoptive family.

When Sandra explains her intentions to the parents, they become angry and threatening. They speak to her in ways which she finds humiliating and deeply upsetting. They challenge the validity of her opinion, the quality of her intellect, the accuracy and even the honesty of her evidence. Jon threatens Sandra with legal action; he tells her that there are other professionals willing to dispute her assessment, the head teacher for example. He threatens to use his powerful connections to ruin her career.

Reflective Exercise 11.1

1 What effect do you think the response from the parents might have upon Sandra's practice?

2 What do you think Sandra should do next?

Six Core Skills in Responding to Resistance

1   Motivational Interviewing: Understanding resistance as 'discord' between individuals and not an inherent quality of the service user (Miller and Rollnick, 2013).

William Miller's early ideas for motivational interviewing arose from his curiosity about the different treatment outcomes achieved by a number of counsellors in the same organisation. The counsellors were all working with service users with alcohol and substance misuse issues. Miller noticed that some counsellors consistently achieved quite astonishingly positive results while, for others, the outcomes were actually worse than if there had been no intervention at all. Miller observed the effectiveness of using an empathic, person-centred style regardless of the initial level of resistance demonstrated by the service users. This observation formed the basis of the motivational interviewing approach which postulates that communication style is a defining factor in service user resistance. So, when professionals meet with resistance, they must ask themselves, 'what do I need to do differently here?'

Miller noted that effective counsellors were able to discover and acknowledge what was important to the service user and hence intrinsically motivating to them. When starting from this point, there was less likelihood of discord.

People struggling to change often experience feelings of ambivalence, for example, 'I know my child needs fresh fruit and I feel really awful, but I need my cigarettes to get through the day without screaming!' This ambivalence can be used to promote change by developing the discrepancy between the current negative behaviour and the positive aspiration and then supporting the individual to make change. (The fact that Peter Connolly's mother frequently took him to her doctor whilst simultaneously disguising his injuries to social workers might have indicated some ambivalence.)

Miller working together with Rollnick used Prochaska and De-Clemente's cycle of change as a framework for their person-centred approach. They included techniques and tools such as the 'readiness ruler' for measuring if a person was 'ready, willing and able' to change and the 'decisional balance' to list and explore the pros and cons of changing or not changing. They promoted a non-confrontational, empathic interaction style of 'rolling with resistance' using reflection of the service users own words to avoid arguments, yet continue to develop discrepancy and 'Motivational Interviewing' was conceptualised. The style is 'collaborative', so congruent with the underpinning principles of partnership working but also 'directive', which is crucially important for safeguarding. Their latest edition offers a simplified intervention structure based on four stages and utilising five key skills:

Engaging: establishing a helpful connection and a working relationship.

Focussing: the process by which you develop and maintain a specific direction in the conversation about change.

Evoking: involves eliciting the client's own motivation for change and lies at the heart of MI.

Planning: developing commitment to change and formulating a concrete plan of action.

Five key communication skills used throughout MI are asking open questions, affirming, reflecting, summarizing and providing information and advice with permission. (Miller and Rollnick, 2013: 32).

Developing discrepancy regarding the abuse of others with individuals who have little empathy for others (for example people with anti-social personality traits) may involve enhancing the individual's 'enlightened self-interest'. This means helping a service user to understand how it is in their own interests to behave pro-socially towards others (NHS, 2012).

2 Developing a trusting, respectful and 'authentic' relationship with the service user.

Smith et al.'s (2011) study of feedback from 'involuntary social work service users' demonstrated the importance of a working relationship characterised by 'trust, honesty, continuity, support and encouragement'. McNeill et al. (2005) found that similar factors enhance service user desistence from offending behaviour:

- accurate empathy, respect or warmth, and therapeutic genuineness;

- establishing a 'therapeutic relationship' or 'working alliance' (mutual understanding and agreement about the nature and purpose of treatment);

- an approach that is person-centred or collaborative and client-driven (taking the client's perspective and using the client's concepts).

(McNeill et al., 2005: 3)

Listening and asking the service user's opinion are immediate demonstrations of respect, so are other behaviours concerned with simple good manners such as punctuality, appropriate dress code, asking people where they would prefer to sit, little things like not taking a cup of tea into a meeting with a service user unless there is a facility to offer one to them too. Using motivational interviewing skills as discussed in stage 1 'engaging' (Miller and Rollnick, 2013) is critical to developing the rapport which enables a relationship to develop. Developing a relationship is the first of three core principles in the highly successful 'Signs of Safety' strengths-based intervention for working towards child protection (Turnell, 2010). There is a wealth of research evidence to support the importance of developing an authentic working relationship with the service user in social work (Munro, 2010; Ruch, 2010).

3   Maintaining clear boundaries with transparent use of professional power.

Service user feedback (Smith et al., 2011) highlights the importance that service users place upon social workers being transparent and honest while holding firm boundaries; exploring options and enabling service user choice where possible but being very clear about the limitations and consequences of those choices and clear where (and why) the social worker may use his or her professional power to impose a course of action. One of the social workers who participated in Smith et al.'s survey expresses this point well:

> I think a lot of our clients feel we are out to get them and if you can turn that around and tell them 'I want to be honest and open' and the way I work is I say to them, 'I am sometimes going to say things to you that you are not going to like . . . but I have to be honest with you [and] if you listen we can try and find a way through it'.
>
> (Smith et al., 2011: 11)

Fauth et al. (2010) in a review of safeguarding practice for the C4EO concluded that:

> Empathy and established relationship skills remain the necessary, but insufficient conditions when working with resistant families; they need to be balanced with an eyes-wide-open, boundaried, authoritative approach aimed at containing anxiety and ensuring that the child's needs stay in sharp focus.
>
> (2)

Ruch (2010) emphasises the point that for social work relationships to be effective, there must be transparency about the power invested in the social worker's role from the outset. There is a parallel with the 'Signs of Safety' second core principle: 'Munro's maxim: thinking critically, fostering a stance of inquiry' (Turnell, 2010: 9). 'Signs of Safety' was developed from years of practitioner wisdom and hinges upon working in partnership with parents and families in child protection.

4   Acknowledging and building upon the service user's strengths.

This can be achieved by exploring exceptions to the problematic behaviour, the strengths in existing support systems and building upon positive constructs which are meaningful and desirable to the service user. Research exploring what service users in the criminal justice system reported had helped them to change demonstrates the significance of being enabled to develop a positive new identity (McNeill, 2006). Research reviewed by Smith et al. (2011) quotes social work service users stressing the value of having their strengths (not just their deficits) recognised by their social workers.

    There have been criticisms of the role of strengths-based approaches in the failure to correctly assess risk. The use of the 'solution focussed brief therapy' model in the case of Peter Connolly highlighted concerns that this model might have caused social workers to lose their focus on risk. However, the serious case review reported that there was

> no evidence from scrutiny of case records or interviews conducted that it had a direct impact on this case or its outcome.

Nevertheless the review stipulated that:

> The SFBT approach has a place in family work and emphasising the strengths of parents is important, but it is not compatible with the authoritative approach to parents in the protective phase of enquiries, assessment and the child protection conference if children are to be protected.
>
> (Haringey LSCB, 2009: 19)

However, strengths-based models such as motivational interviewing (Miller and Rollnick, 2013) and solution-focused brief therapy (Kondrat in Teater, 2014) if used properly, do stress the importance of practitioners only ever giving authentic feedback to service users for specific positive actions. NHS (2012) guidelines on working with personality disordered service users advise that 'tangible evidence' of positive behaviour should be observed rather simply taking the word of the service user. The 'Signs of Safety' model, as previously mentioned, provides a successful strengths-based intervention model in child protection (Turnell, 2010).

5   Seeking supervision for reflection, assessment, support and self-esteem.

There is a wealth of evidence from every enquiry and study of serious case reviews to support the necessity of supportive supervision as a forum for reflective practice and sound decision making (Brandon et al., 2009; Ruch et al., 2010). Laird (2013a) maintains that 'self-esteem' is a necessary requirement of assertive professional practice. Social work educators and managers should take care to create supportive learning environments which present manageable challenges thus fostering confidence. Laird provides a case study discussion of when a social worker becomes isolated as a consequence of unsupportive supervision and hence susceptible to identifying with a manipulative and hostile service user (Laird, 2013a: 123–140). Social workers must take responsibility for seeking supervision and peer support when they are wrestling with difficult emotions (Urdang, 2010). Organisations which foster peer case discussions tend to make better assessments (Munro, 2010; Turnell, 2010).

6   Practising de-escalation micro-skills.

Laird (2013) argues for the importance of practitioners being able to use de-escalation skills to assist in the development of professional assertiveness.

The implication is that the way a worker behaves can have an impact on the levels of aggression used by the service user. This message is evident in research with mental health service users where:

> the attitudes and behaviour of staff have been found to be the most important factors affecting patients' aggressive behaviour.
>
> (Abderhalden et al. 2006 in Holmes et al. 2012: 3)

and also when working with aggression in a prison setting where:

> It has always been recognised that the best defensive weapon that staff have is their verbal and non-verbal communication skills. Staff who successfully adopt effective communication strategies ... and interpersonal skills will find that they are usually able to defuse a potential conflict.
>
> (HMPS, 2005: 7)

Forrester et al.'s (2008) study of the communication style of 40 social workers found that the majority tended to use a confrontational and at times aggressive approach in simulated child protection interviews. The study concluded that the teaching of relevant micro-skills was an urgent priority.

Taylor (2011) makes the point that the social workers best able to de-escalate aggression rarely have to deal with any. The implications here for reducing stress and 'burn-out' and supporting professional resilience are clear.

Oliver (2006) suggests that practitioner mood and perspective are crucial in de-escalating angry people. She suggests that (if there is a choice in the matter) practitioners should ask themselves 'am I in the proper frame of mind to handle an angry person?' 'Can I view them as someone who is doing what they can to get their needs met?'

Box 11.1 **Practice skill outline: 'de-escalation'**

Do you recognise the non-verbal signals of escalation in others?

- Standing tall
- Raised voice
- Rapid breathing
- Direct prolonged eye contact
- Exaggerated gestures

Are you aware of your own body language? Try the following:

- Adopt a non-threatening body posture
- Reduce direct eye contact (as it may be taken as a confrontation)
- Allow the person adequate personal space
- Keep both hands visible
- Avoid sudden movements
- Stand at a 45 degree angle to the person.

Practise the following six communication techniques.

1 SIMPLE LISTENING

- Sometimes all that is needed is to allow the angry person to vent all their anger and frustration to someone who actually listens.
- Listen attentively, nod your head and sometimes encourage using terms such as 'Uh- huh', 'Go on' or 'Yes'.
- Listen until their anger is spent. At that point you could ask a simple question such as, 'Is there anything I can do to help?'

2 ACTIVE LISTENING

- Active listening is the empathic process of really attempting to understand and acknowledge what a person is saying.
- If you try a reflection of feeling, do so very cautiously in case you have got it wrong! 'I'm guessing you feel…'
- Give the person the opportunity to correct you. 'Have I got that right?'

3 RESPECTFUL ACKNOWLEDGEMENT

- Acknowledgement occurs when we can genuinely understand the person's angry emotion. You could then honestly respond with, 'I can see how that would make you angry!'
- Tone of voice is critical in this circumstance. An excitable tone could further incite more angry behaviour – use a calming and respectful tone, as if you were speaking to a colleague or business associate.

4 APOLOGISING

- Not for an imaginary wrong, but sincerely apologising for anything in the situation that you believe was unfair. A simple statement acknowledging that something occurred that wasn't right.

◀

- If you can't find anything to sincerely apologise about, you can say, 'I'm sorry you are having such an awful time'. You can apologise without taking on the blame.

5 AGREEING

- Often when people are angry about something, there is at least 2 per cent of truth in what they are saying.
- It is important to listen for that 2 per cent of truth and agree with it.

6 INVITING CRITICISM

- Simply ask the angry person to voice his or her criticism of us or the situation more fully. You may say something like 'Go ahead. Tell me everything that has upset you'.

When nothing works, remember the following:

- safety should be the primary concern;
- never get between the angry person and his or her only means of escape;
- never allow the angry person to block your only means of escape;
- try to close the discussion and lead the person towards the exit.

Develop an agency approach:

- efforts that are successful in minimising danger are rarely solo acts;
- be aware of procedures for obtaining assistance from other staff members;
- using whatever is available to create loud noise or call attention to an area;
- initiating a predetermined signal/panic alarm or scratch of the head;
- conduct joint home visits and co-work difficult cases.

Adapted from Oliver (2006) and HMPS (2005).

Conclusion

Of course there are no quick fixes to working with resistance and particularly in safeguarding contexts where service users often experience social workers as powerful persecutory figures intervening in their private lives. However, it is working with this particular tension between care and control which characterises the social work profession perhaps more than any other. Arguably there is no inherent ethical conflict, especially not in the safeguarding role, if the worker retains a clear focus on their task of protecting a child or adult at risk. The relationship with the parent or carer must be built around that premise. Evidence from a number of professional perspectives including health, criminal justice, social work and service user feedback indicates that there is a core micro-skill set which is critical for working with all forms of resistance. The good news is that it is a refinement of the same skill set required for good communication with voluntary service users. In safeguarding situations, the skill set may at first appear to have contradictions such as 'empowerment' and 'transparent use of authority'. It requires expertise, professional capability and confidence to be effective but there is no contradiction if the professional intention is clear. Social workers must understand how to 'roll with resistance'; they must not confuse the need for clear professional boundaries with using a confrontational approach, nor must they confuse compassionate responses to abusive parents and carers with failure to protect children and adults at risk. Rather they must develop the skills to manage clear boundaries whilst demonstrating compassion, they should be able to discover what is most important in the mind of the parent in order to protect the child, and even if things do escalate, the required skill set still involves listening, acknowledging, empathising and affirming.

The discussion above is intended to demonstrate how motivational interviewing skills as part of an overarching strengths-based approach can assist the social work student and practitioner to build a relationship within which the social worker has permission to ask to 'look inside the food cupboard' without experiencing role conflict or breaching the expectations of the service user. The caring relationship is built solidly around shared knowledge of the power imbalance not flimsily by blurring boundaries or pretending that the imbalance does not exist.

Joseph and Benefield's useful list of skills required for working with offenders who have a personality disorder can be applied generally to most forms of social work practice. These skills are as follows:

- a capacity to maintain boundaries whilst also being flexible and responsive;
- emotional maturity and personal resilience;
- a capacity to empower the service user;
- maintenance of a positive attitude and an acceptance of what is (and is not) possible;
- capacity for reflection and willingness to be open about uncertainties;
- capacity for team and shared working;
- positive and rewarding approaches are more likely to be effective in engaging and keeping people in services than negative and punitive ones.

(Joseph and Benefield, 2012: 71)

By learning how to establish caring, professional and transparent relationships and accessing supervision and support, social workers will reduce both the occurrence and negative impact of hostile and manipulative responses from service users. This approach will enhance the workers emotional resilience, the quality of their assessments and the outcomes for service users, carers and children and adults at risk.

Reflective Exercise 11.2 **Considering 'discord' and resistance**

1 Identify a situation in your practice when you experienced or perceived resistance from a service user.

2 Considering the ideas in the discussion above, what do you think may have been the reason for the resistance you encountered?

3 Is there anything you would have done differently if applying the six skills above?

Case study 11:2 **Lena and her family (part 2)**

Sandra listens to the threats and accusations. She avoids defending herself or contradicting the hostile parents. She agrees to take their concerns to her manager re-affirming that any decisions will be made in the children's best interests. Sandra then seeks out her manager and explains to him exactly what is happening. She describes her concerns for Lena and the other children; she describes her preoccupation with the case, her doubts about her assessment, her sleeplessness and her fear of losing her career. Her manager listens and explores the evidence recorded in the file. He supports Sandra's assessment and the decision to remove Lena from her parents care. He directs Sandra to the agency legal team. He also reduces the number of cases Sandra is holding and suggests that she speaks to a colleague in another team who worked with the family previously.

Following a family court hearing, Lena goes directly from school to a foster family. Her behaviour improves immediately and she settles well.

Social work involvement with the family continues with a new social worker, Frances, from the Children Looked After team. Frances arranges to meet Mel alone. She shares with Mel that Lena is settling well. She allows Mel time to reflect on this. Mel acknowledges that perhaps there were things she might have done differently. Frances listens as Mel describes her feelings of anger, loss and regret and fear of losing the love and custody of her sons.

Mel: 'I really wanted to be that "Mother-Earth-Superstar" you know? To have "rescued these children" and to be so much better than my mother was to me.'

Frances: 'Better than your mother was to you?'

Mel: 'I don't want to talk about that, but my mother was … impossible; it's complicated; but I really wanted to do better.'

▶

Frances: 'Do you think because you wanted so much to be a good mum, it was too painful to see your behaviour as part of the problem?'

Mel: [Pauses] 'Yes ... I think so, but not just that ... it was Jon's career too. We couldn't be seen as incompetent in any way; and Lena behaved so terribly, she just was the problem in our eyes.'

Frances: 'So you felt under pressure to give the impression that you were this "perfect family" because of Jon's career status? That must have been tough.'

Mother: 'Yes, it sounds shallow, but there was so much pressure. Jon would get hysterical if Lena played up; I know you can't imagine it when you see him ... but he would! I totally panicked when I couldn't control her. I half-knew deep down it was my mess but I couldn't admit it, I kept hoping it would work out somehow. It was driving me crazy and I was ... I was really horrible to Lena.'

Reflective Exercise 11.3 **Considering motivation**

- What do you think were the critical factors which enabled Sandra to resist the threats?
- Why do you think Mel shares her vulnerability with Frances more than she did with Sandra?
- Where do you think Mel is on the cycle of change?
- What are your thoughts about working with Jon?

Progress Check

The professional capability framework for social workers 'PCF' (TCSW 2012) is a holistic framework and hence most domains will apply simultaneously to any given example of good social work practice. The PCF domains and the Health and Care Professions Council standards of proficiency 'HCPC SoPs' HCPC (2012) listed below are those which relate most directly to this chapter and which encompass the complexity and apparent contradictions of care and control particularly apparent when assessing and intervening with families.

PCF 7.3 Demonstrate the ability to engage with people, and build, manage, sustain and conclude compassionate and effective relationships.

PCF 7.12 Recognise the factors that create or exacerbate risk to individuals, their families or carers, to the public or to professionals, including yourself, and contribute to the assessment and management of risk.

HCPC SoP 8.4 Understand how communication skills affect the assessment of and engagement with service users and carers.

HCPC SoP 8.6 Be aware of the characteristics and consequences of verbal and non-verbal communication and how this can be affected by a range of factors including age, culture, disability, ethnicity, gender, religious beliefs and socio-economic status.

PCF 6.4 Demonstrate a capacity for logical, systematic, critical and reflective reasoning and apply the theories and techniques of reflective practice.

HCPC SoP 11.1 Understand the value of critical reflection on practice and the need to record the outcome of such reflection appropriately.

Consider how you feel your practice is developing with regard to these PCF domains and SoPs. There may be issues here which you wish to discuss in supervision and/or which highlight further training needs for you.

Chapter Summary

- Working with resistance is an everyday aspect of professional social work and particularly when working with safeguarding issues.

- Working with resistance involves understanding different presentations and possible underlying causes.

- Social workers and students must be self-aware in terms of their values, theoretical perspectives and actions with regard to the impact their behaviour has in fuelling or reducing service user resistance.

- Social workers and students should practise motivational micro-skills in communication to develop meaningful working relationships with service users.

- Social workers and students should be able to access the support of their managers and colleagues in order to avoid isolation and develop the confidence to report power and control tactics of service users using threats and aggression.

- Social workers and students must be exceptionally clear with service users about the power, authority and responsibilities of their role and develop an honest and caring rapport which acknowledges this duality from the outset.

Further Reading

- Hohman, M. (2012) *Motivational Interviewing in Social Work Practice.* New York: Guilford Press.

  This book presents motivational interviewing concepts with specific consideration of their application in social work.

- Laird S. E. (2013) *Child Protection, Managing Conflict Hostility and Aggression*. Bristol: The Policy Press.

  This book provides an analysis of issues involving conflict and aggression in child protection work. It is filled with interesting case studies and recent research.

- Miller, W. R. and Rollnick, S. (2013) *Motivational Interviewing: Helping People Change*. New York: Guilford Press.

  This is the latest work from Miller and Rollnick, the founding fathers of Motivational Interviewing, and contains updated ideas for use in varied practice contexts.

- Turnell, A. (2010) The Signs of Safety; A Comprehensive Briefing Paper, available at http://www.peterboroughlscb.org.uk/files/Signs of safety briefing paper v1-031.pdf

  Provides a concise account of the development and application of the Signs of Safety Model.

References

Abderhalden, C., Hahn, S., Bonner, Y.D.B., Galeazzi, G.M. (2006) Users' Perceptions and Views on Violence and Coercion in Mental Health. In: Richter, D., Whittington, D. (eds), *Violence in Mental Health Settings: Causes, Consequences, Management*. New York: Springer. In Holmes, D., Rudge, T., Perron, A. and St Pierre, I. (2012) *(Re) Thinking Violence in Health Care Settings*. Farnham: Ashgate.

Bandura, A. (1977) *Social Learning Theory*. Englewood Cliffs, NJ: Prentice Hall. In Teater B. (ed.) (2014) *An Introduction to Applying Social Work Theories and Methods*. Berkshire: Open University Press.

Brandon, M., Bailey, S., Belderson, P., Gardner, R., Sidebotham, P., Dodsworth, J., Warren, C. and Black, J. (2009) Understanding Serious Case Reviews and Their Impact: A Biennial Analysis of Serious Case Reviews 2005–07, London (Research report No DCSF-RR129) London: DCSF, available at https://www.google.co.uk/webhp?sourceid=chrome-instant&rlz=1C1ARAB_enGB456GB456&ion=1&espv=2&ie=UTF-8#, accessed 19 June 2014.

Cleaver, H., Unwell, I. and Aldgate J. (2011) *Children's Needs Parenting Capacity*, 2nd edition. London: The Stationery Office.

Craissati, J., Chuan, S. J., Simons, S. and Joseph, N. (2011) *Working with Personality Disordered Offenders: A Practitioner's Guide*. Oxleas NHS Foundation, available at http://www.justice.gov.uk/downloads/offenders/mentally-disordered-offenders/working-with-personality-disordered-offenders.pdf, accessed 26 June 2014.

DCSF (2007) Engaging Effectively with Black and Minority Ethnic Parents in Children's and Parental Services, available at http://www.education.gov.uk/publications/RSG/publicationDetail/Page1/DCSF-RR013, accessed 26 June 2014.

Fauth, B., Jelicic, H., Hart, D. and Burton, S. (2010). Effective Practice to Protect Children Living in 'Highly Resistant' Families. Centre for Excellence and Outcomes in Children and Young People's Services (C4EO), available at http://www.c4eo.org.uk/evidence/default.aspx, accessed 26 June 2014.

Forrester, D., Kershaw, S., Moss, H. and Hughes, L. (2008) Communication Skills in Child Protection: How Do Social Workers Talk to Parents? *Child and Family Social Work*, 13: 41–51, available at http://onlinelibrary.wiley.com/doi/10.1111/j.1365-2206.2007.00513, accessed 19 June 2014.

Gast, L. and Patmore, A. (2012) *Mastering Approaches to Diversity in Social Work*. London: Jessica Kingsley.

Haringey LSCB (2009) Serious Case Review Baby Peter, available at http://www.haringeylscb.org/executive_summary_peter_final.pdf, accessed 26 June 2014.

HCPC (2012) *Standards of Proficiency*. Health and Care Professions Council: Publication code: 20120521POLPUB.

Hester, M. (2011) The Three Planet Model: Towards an Understanding of Contradictions in Approaches to Women and Children's Safety in Contexts of Domestic Violence, *British Journal of Social Work*, 41: 837–853.

HM Government (2013) Working Together to Safeguard Children: A Guide to Inter-agency Working to Safeguard and Promote the Welfare of Children, available at http://www.workingtogetheronline.co.uk/documents/Working%20TogetherFINAL.pdf, accessed 25 June 2014.

HMPS (2005) Use of Force: Prison service order number 1600, available at https://www.justice.gov.uk/downloads/offenders/psipso/pso/pso-1600.doc, accessed 19 June 2014.

Hohman, M. (2012) *Motivational Interviewing in Social Work Practice*. New York: The Guilford Press.

Holmes, D., Rudge, T., Perron, A. and St Pierre, I. (2012) *(Re) Thinking Violence in Health Care Settings*. Farnham: Ashgate.

Howe D. (1995) Attachment Theory and Social Work Practice London: Palgrave Macmillan.

Joseph, N. and Benefield, N. (2012) *The Offender Personality Disorder Strategy Commissioning the Pathway*. Department of Health/NOMS personality disorder policy team, available at http://www.probationchiefs.org/uploads/newsletters/pca/pca/pd Workshop- 12th April 2012.pdf, accessed 25 June 2014.

Joseph Rowntree Foundation, available at http://www.jrf.org.uk/publications/young-disabled-people-moving-adulthood-scotland, accessed 6 July 2014.

Kenny, L. and Kenny, B. (2000) Psychodynamic Theory in Social Work: A View from Practice. In Stepney, P. and Ford, D. (eds), *Social Work Models Methods and Theories*. Lyme Regis: Russell House.

Kondrat, D. C. Solution Focussed Practice. In Teater B. (ed.) (2014) *An Introduction to Applying Social Work Theories and Methods*, 2nd edition. Berkshire: Open University Press.

Laird, S. E. (2013) Training Social Workers to Effectively Manage Aggressive Parental Behaviour in Child Protection in Australia, the United States and the United Kingdom, *British Journal of Social Work*, doi:10.1093/bjsw/bct043, 1–17, available at http://bjsw.oxfordjournals.org/content/early/2013/03/10/bjsw.bct043.full.pdf, accessed 26 June 2014.

Laird, S. E. (2013a) *Child Protection: Managing Conflict Hostility and Aggression*. Bristol: The Policy Press.

Laming, H. (2003) *The Victoria Climbié Inquiry Report*. London: The Stationery Office, available at www.dh.gov.uk/en/Publicationsandstatistics/Publications/Publications PolicyAndGuidance/DH_4008654, accessed 26 June 2014.

LGA (2013) Adult Safeguarding and Domestic Abuse: A Guide to Support Practitioners and Managers, available at http://www.local.gov.uk/publications//journal_content/56/10180/3973717/PUBLICATION, accessed 26 June 2014.

Littlechild, B. (2005) The Nature and Effects of Violence against Child-Protection Social Workers: Providing Effective Support, *British Journal of Social Work*, 35: 387–401.

LSCB Haringey. (2009) Serious case Review: Baby Peter. Executive Summary, available at http://www.haringeylscb.org/executive_summary_peter_final.pdf, accessed 26 June 2014.

Mason, R. (2014) Available at http://www.theguardian.com/society/2014/mar/03/female-genital-mutilation-law-police-acpo-fgm-parents-cutters, accessed 6 July 2014.

McNeill, F. (2006) A Desistance Paradigm for Offender Management, *Criminology and Criminal Justice*, 6 (1): 39–62, available at http://crj.sagepub.com/content/6/1/39, accessed 14 June 2014.

McNeill, F. (2009) What Works and What's Just? *European Journal of Probation*, 1 (1): 21–40, available at https://pure.strath.ac.uk/...works-and-whats-just(e9305732.../export.html, accessed 12 June 2014.

McNeill, F., Batchelor, S., Burnett, R. and Knox, J. (2005) *Reducing Re-Offending – Key Practice Skills, 21st Century Social Work*. Edinburgh: Scottish Executive, available at http://www.scotland.gov.uk/Resource/Doc/37432/0011296.pdf, accessed 26 June 2014.

Miller, W. R. and Rollnick, S. (2013) *Motivational Interviewing: Helping People Change*. New York: Guilford Press.

Monds-Watson, A. (2011) Understanding Aggression and Resistance. In Taylor B. J. (ed.) *Working with Aggression and Resistance in Social Work*. Exeter: Learning Matters.

Munro, E. (2010) *The Munro Review of Child Protection Part One: A Systems Analysis*. London: Crown Copyright, available at https://www.gov.uk/government/uploads/system/uploads/attachment_data/file/175407/TheMunroReview-Part_one.pdf, accessed 6 July 2014.

Narey, M. (2014) Making the Education of Social Workers Consistently Effective: Report of Sir Martin Narey's Independent Review of the Education of Children's Social Workers, available at https://www.gov.uk/government/uploads/system/uploads/attachment_data/file/287756/Making_the_education_of_social_workers_consistently_effective.pdf, accessed 25 June 2014.

NHS (2012) *Working to Enable and Empower Front Line Staff to Work More Effectively with Offenders with Personality Disorder*. The Impact Team: Camden and Islington, available at http://www.candi.nhs.uk/_uploads/documents/impact/impact-newsletter-may-2012.pdf, accessed 25 June 2014.

Oliver, K. (2006) De-escalation Techniques: How to Take the Wind out of their Sails, available at http://www.articlesbase.com/self-help-articles/deescalation-techniques-how-to-take-the-wind-out-of-their-sails-92797.html, accessed 19 June 2014.

Perry, B. D. (2005) Inaugural Lecture, Maltreatment and the Developing Child: How Early Childhood Experience Shapes Child and Culture: Centre for Children and Families in the Justice System, available at www.lfcc.on.ca/mccain/perry.pdf, accessed 6 July 2014.

Phillips, A. (2010) *Gender and Culture*. Cambridge: Polity Press.

Prochaska, J. O. and Di Clemente, C. C. (2005) The Transtheoretical Approach. In: Norcross, J. C. and Goldfried, M. R. (eds), *Handbook of Psychotherapy Integration*, 2nd edition, 147–171. London: Oxford University Press.

Reder, P., Duncan, S. and Gray, M. (1993) *Beyond Blame: Child Abuse Tragedies Revisited.* London: Routledge.

Renteln, A. D. (2010) Corporal Punishment and the Cultural Defence, *Journal of Law and Contemporary Problems*, 73: 253–279, available at http://scholarship.law.duke.edu/lcp/vol73/iss2/10, accessed 6 July 2014.

Ruch, G. (2010) The Contemporary Context of Relationship-Based Practice. In: Ruch, G., Turney, D. and Ward, A. (eds). *Relationship-Based Social Work*. London: Jessica Kingsley Publications.

Scott, K. (2010) Caring Dads Theory Manual, available at http://caringdads.org/pros/res/ap/131-caring-dads-theory-manual, accessed 6 July 2014.

Sheldon, B. (2000) Cognitive Behavioural Methods in Social Care: A Look at the Evidence. In: Stepney, P. and Ford, D. (eds), *Social Work Models Methods and Theories*. Lyme Regis: Russell House Publishing.

Smith, M. (2005) *Surviving Fears in Health and Social Care*. London: Jessica Kingsley.

Smith, M., Gallagher, M., Wosu, H., Stewart, J., Cree, V. E., Hunter, S., Evans, S., Montgomery, C., Holiday, S. and Wilkinson H. (2011) Engaging with Involuntary Service Users in Social Work: Findings from a Knowledge Exchange Project, *British Journal of Social Work*, 162: 1–18, available at www.socialwork.ed.ac.uk/people/academic_staff/smith_mark, accessed 6 July 2014.

Stanley, J. and Goddard, C. (2002) *In the Firing Line: Violence and Power in Child Protection Work*. Chichester: Wiley.

Stanley, N. (2011) *Children Experiencing Domestic Violence: A Research Review*. Dartington: Research in Practice.

Stobart, E. (2009) Multi-Agency Practice Guidelines: Handling Cases of Forced Marriage, available at https://www.gov.uk/government/.../forced-marriage-guidelines09, accessed 6 July 2014.

Taylor, B. J. (2011) Avoiding Assault and Diffusing Aggression. In Taylor, B. J. (ed.), *Working with Aggression and Resistance in Social Work*. Exeter: Learning Matters.

TCSW (2012) The Professional Capabilities Framework (P. C. F.) Available at http://www.tcsw.org.uk/pcf.aspx, accessed 26 June 2014.

Teater, B. (2014) *An Introduction To Applying Social Work Theories And Methods*, 2nd edition. Berkshire: Open University Press.

Turnell, A. (2010) The Signs of Safety; A Comprehensive Briefing Paper, available at http://www.peterboroughlscb.org.uk/files/Signs of safety briefing paper v1-031.pdf, accessed 6 July 2014.

Ward, A. (2010) The Use of Self in Relationship-Based Practice. In Ruch, G., Turney, D. and Ward, A. (eds) *Relationship-Based Social Work*. London: Jessica Kingsley Publications.

Webster-Stratton, C. (1998) *Parent Training with Low income Families: Handbook of Child Abuse Research and Treatment*. New York: Plenum Press.

Urdang, E. (2010) Awareness of Self: A Critical Tool, *Social Work Education*, 29 (5): 523–538, available at http://www.bu.edu/ssw/files/2010/10/Awareness-of-Self-A-Critical-Tool.pdf, accessed 15 June 2014.

YJB (2011) Engaging Service Users: Barriers and Enablers, available at http://www.justice.gov.uk/downloads/youth-justice/yjb-toolkits/parenting/engaging-service-users.pdf, accessed 26 June 2014.

INDEX